A Migraine In Room 3, A Stroke In Room 4

A Physician Examines His Profession

Paul M. Schanfield, MD

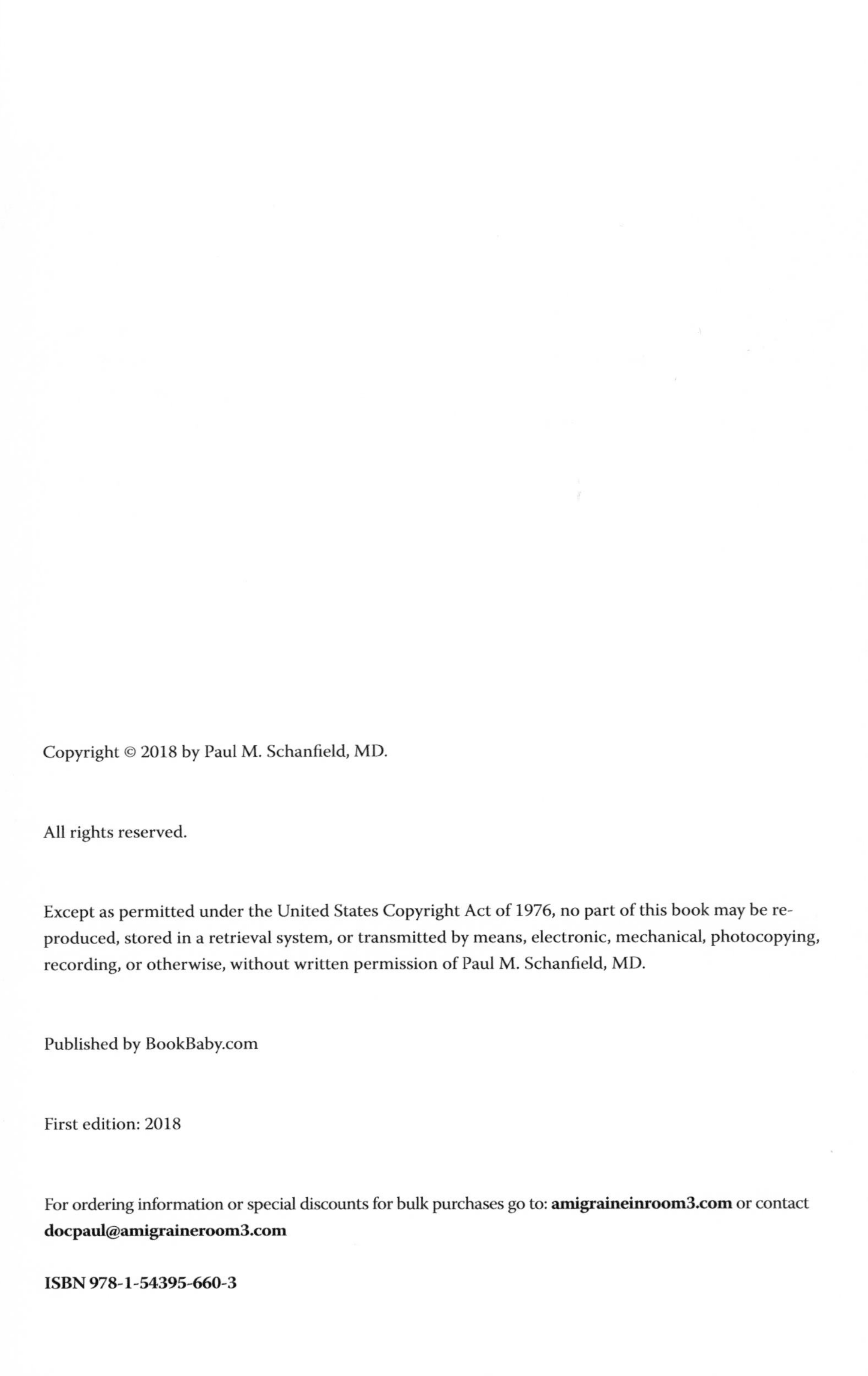

Published by BookBaby.com

First edition: 2018

For ordering information or special discounts for bulk purchases go to: **amigraineinroom3.com** or contact **docpaul@amigraineroom3.com**

ISBN 978-1-54395-660-3

DEDICATION

My career choice of medicine grew primarily from my desire to help people in need. Throughout my career, my life was enriched by the joy of listening, laughing, and crying with my patients. As I accompanied them and their families facing disease, disability, and death, they taught me invaluable lessons about life, illness, and aging. Their stories represent sad, ingenious, humorous, and hopeful examples of human resilience in the face of life crises.

My patients made the long and grueling hours of work worthwhile, facilitating my love of practicing medicine. They motivated me to chronicle their stories. I hope this book honors their lives.

FOREWORD

"What does your father do?" When I was younger, I always dreaded this question. Not because I wasn't impressed by and proud of my father. It was the predictable follow up questions that would inevitably present themselves that I always tried to sidestep. When dancing around the question was no longer polite, I'd inhale and quickly mumble:

> "Well, my dad is a doctor."
> "What kind of doctor?"
> "A neurologist."
> "Oh, cool, a brain surgeon!"
> "Um, no, he doesn't do surgery."
> "Oh, so what does your mom do?"

Being a neurologist meant my dad worked a lot. Nights. Weekends. Early mornings. While he worked late and often missed time with the family on both ends of the day, surprisingly his absence does not punctuate my childhood memories. Instead, I remember his presence.

He usually left for work well before my brother Adam and I rolled out of bed. My dad had a special way of letting us know that we mattered to him. He'd scrawl a greeting on whatever colorful drug-company branded post-it pad he could find (my favorite was the giant ones shaped like brains!). The note would contain a word puzzle, treasure hunt (find the note under the "place where you steal things from," aka cookie jar), clever pun, a classic dad joke, or just a simple "love you - see you later!" The notes were there to start the day...his unique way of being present. If I had been wise enough to save them, this book would contain a lengthy appendix.

During my high school athletics days, I'm not sure he ever heard the national anthem or the starting lineup announced, but he always showed up eventually. His effort to attend games was one way I learned how much showing up really matters. For someone dealing with end of life decisions all day and pacing the ICU by night, my father still found the time and energy to cheer me on.

At the end of the day, my dad made great efforts to show up at home in time for dinner, even if it meant he'd come home to eat with us and return to the office. Those dinners nearly always began in a predictable fashion, with my dad saying, "So...I saw this little old lady in the office today...."

He would then reach into his breast pocket and pull out his rounds card with copious scribbles on both sides, in every direction. He would flip it over a few times, look at it, squint to try to read his own handwriting, smile, and recount patient encounters from earlier that day, complete with a nasally voice over for dramatic effect. The stories ranged from sweet to silly to tragic. Sometimes it was a funny response to "How are you feeling today?" ("Aren't I paying you to tell me that, doc?"), or a vivid description of a headache ("It feels like a fat old lady standing on my eyeballs in high heels."). It filled him with infinite delight to share those stories with us. He cared for his patients with a personal and honest flare for over four decades, and they reciprocated by sharing their personal stories with him.

As it turns out, my dad had been stuffing those patient quotes and stories into a shoebox...almost every day. One day in 2015, when retirement loomed, he opened the shoebox and began to type. Some 75 pages later, he had the makings of a book. Under the tutelage of Paul Bernabei, an author, esteemed educator, and friend-turned-writing coach, he now shares those stories. In this book, he examines the healthcare system from multiple angles, spells out his theories on medical education, and concludes with his prescription for dealing with the current healthcare crisis.

"So what does my father do?"

My father shows up. He has made a medical career of being with his patients. He sits with you, listens to you, jokes with you, and always answers phone calls. He cares about what you have to say, and he is there when you need him.

And now, dear reader, it's your turn to have a man I am proud to call "Dad" show up and say, "So I saw this little old lady in the office today...."

Mara Schanfield

"The good physician treats the disease;
the great physician treats the patient who has the disease."

—William Osler

TABLE OF CONTENTS

PREFACE

Welcome to the story of one physician's 40-year career, predicated on treating patients as people with medical problems, concerns, or anxieties rather than as medical problems in business-style healthcare. Physicians do not treat migraines. Physicians do not treat strokes. Physicians treat *people* with migraines and *individuals* who have suffered strokes.

While this story started as an autobiography, it evolved into a multidimensional undertaking. The practice of clinical medicine is based fundamentally on the art of listening to people in need. A physician listens to people, translating what they say into the language of medicine. The final step in this process is for the physician to successfully convey information to the patient and family in language they understand. When it comes to the most reliable means of formulating an accurate diagnosis and an appropriate treatment plan, no substitute exists for this person-to-person process.

Besides successfully reaching accurate diagnoses and instituting suitable treatment plans, the art of empathetic listening facilitates the opportunity for patients to teach their physician invaluable life lessons. It is my privilege to pass the lessons taught to me on to the reader.

In addition to giving voice to my patients, it is my hope that my story will be instructive for medical students, residents, and fellows. It is my hope these trainees will find the philosophy of medical practice and medical education spelled out in these pages valuable and enlightening. It is my hope that this book will enhance their enjoyment of their chosen profession, while providing tools to prevent today's rampant curse of professional burnout.

This story begins with my description of how the modern medical care model contributes to today's American healthcare crisis by subordinating the physician-patient contract, as spelled out clearly in the Hippocratic Oath, to the business of providing healthcare. My plea is to resurrect the primacy of the fundamental physician-patient contract over the current all-consuming focus on the process, returning the patient to the center of the system. It is my hope that this narrative will educate and interest people from all walks of life, especially those who may have the power to effect the changes needed.

> *"Where there is love of medicine, there is love of humankind."*
> *—Hippocrates*

My Story

The career path to becoming a physician was long and arduous. My path was no exception. My college experience began in 1965 as a College of Liberal Arts pre-med student at the University of Minnesota. The 1960s was an era of social upheaval and heightened sensitivity to justice and equality. As premedical students, my friends and I were not pursuing prestige or money. We were motivated to help others and were fascinated by the sciences, rarely shying away from hard work. We wanted to make a difference. We described ourselves as "people persons," determined to become physicians to help patients regain their health, stay healthy, or cope with illness, life, and death.

We wanted to interact with patients as human beings, not as vessels of disease presenting problems to be solved. We envisioned ourselves practicing medicine as humanely and kindly as possible, while providing the highest quality care. We were young, idealistic, and confident.

My fellow medical students came from varied backgrounds. One had been a University of Minnesota football player who played in the Rose Bowl, was drafted into the army, and served as a medic in Vietnam. One was a lab technician who went to medical school after she realized that the doctors ordering the lab tests seemed no smarter than she was.

Although we did not realize it at the time, as individuals who were primarily motivated to help others and prepared to work long hours, we were more likely to experience long-term satisfaction with less professional "burnout" than if we were in pursuit of money, prestige, or work/life balance. We endeavored to establish personal connections with our patients, empowering our patients to educate us about life, family, disability, aging, and death.

By practicing medicine in this way, we envisioned remaining with our patients over the long term, little realizing that this promise would become less the norm as time passed. Yet, I believe the foundation we built our expectations upon improved treatment success, enhanced patient and physician satisfaction, and lessened patient suffering.

After finishing my pre-med courses, I spent the next eight years in medical training, spanning medical school, an internship, and a neurology residency. From the completion of training in 1976 until my retirement at the end of 2015, I was a private practice neurologist in St. Paul, Minnesota.

Why Neurology?

> ***"I am of the opinion that the brain exercises the greatest power in the man."***
> ***—Hippocrates***

Despite favoring primary care, I was introduced to neurology early in my collegiate life. While still an undergraduate student, I was hired as a clinical research assistant during the summer by Joseph A. Resch, MD, Vice Chairman of the Neurology Department at the University of Minnesota. He helped me organize and publish in a meaningful way a small portion of the data from the department's joint, long-standing Japanese-American Stroke Study.

While working that summer in the Neurology Department, it was easy for me to attend weekly medical student neurology lectures, which I loved. Early in my career, the clinical relevance of neurology was crystallized for me.

How fortunate for me that, as the years went by, I discovered that neurology was indeed a good "fit" for my skill set. Neurology is the study of diseases of the nervous system with widespread consequences anywhere in body, often leading to chronic maladies which allowed me to follow patients for years.

The nervous system is anatomically, chemically, and physiologically complex, which explains why the mastery of it is intellectually challenging. This complexity discourages many medical students from considering the neurosciences as a profession. The brain is still referred to as the last relatively unexplored frontier on earth. The wealth of information to be learned and investigated in the neurosciences can easily consume multiple lifetimes of the best and the brightest.

As a third-year medical student, I was, at times, drawn to other fields of medical discipline that seemed easy, enjoyable, and rewarding. To experience the joy and miracle of the birth of a healthy baby cannot be overstated. In contrast, as a neurologist, dealing with a child with life-threatening bacterial meningitis or head trauma can be trying and frightening.

As medical school progressed, I realized that laboratory, microscope work, and research would not provide me with enough patient contact. I realized that my aptitudes were not visual-spatial, so surgery and radiology seemed unwise choices. I enjoyed and wanted to interact with adults and children, men and women.

However, I did briefly consider neurosurgery. With my intense interest and advanced knowledge of neuroscience, the neurosurgery chief resident allowed me to do a surgical case as a senior med student, albeit under his careful supervision. I came out of the surgery thrilled and pleased with my performance. However, in the surgical locker room, I was stunned to find the neurosurgery chief resident soaked with sweat. I looked at him. He looked at me, shook his head, and said one word to me, "Neurology." That moment ended my consideration of a surgical career, for which I am eternally grateful.

Imagine the wonder of considering why a stroke victim can write but not read. Imagine the wonder of considering why a woman cannot see to the left, yet does not realize the left half of her visual field is missing. Imagine the drama involved when deciding a hole must be drilled into a man's head immediately after he lapses into a coma right in front of you. Imagine being able to stop a person from having one seizure after another.

When I compared such complex maladies with episodes of vomiting blood, diarrhea, wheezing, identifying a rash, or characterizing a heart murmur, the appeal of neurology was compelling and it has continued to be so throughout my professional life. My continued curiosity with the functioning of the brain and the complexity of the nervous system won out. The hardship and challenge of specializing in the neurosciences turned out to be worth the effort of conquering such a difficult body of information.

Besides the complexity of the nervous system, some medical students don't consider neurology because of our limited ability to "fix things." When my daughter considered a career in medicine, I sent her to shadow an accomplished neurosurgeon at the University of Minnesota medical center. When asked if she would consider neurology, she replied that she might. With a grin, the neurosurgeon explained that he could easily and quickly teach her to function as a neurologist. When faced with a patient with a neurological problem, the typical neurologist, he explained, would cross her arms across her chest, tip the head to one side, and say, "Hmm, isn't that an interesting dilemma?"

Yet, during my professional career, I have been fortunate to witness dramatic diagnostic and treatment breakthroughs. Marvelous new tools to image and study the brain and the nervous system have been perfected. These tools have revealed many of the secrets of the nervous system, increasing my fascination with neurology.

In the mid-1970s, the cause of Multiple Sclerosis (MS) was unknown with no FDA-approved treatment. We now understand the patho-physiology of MS and have 15 FDA-approved medications. The introduction of Levo-dopa to replace the missing brain neurotransmitter in Parkinson's Disease became clinically useful in the 1970s, significantly improving the lives of thousands. When I was in training, only a handful of medications existed to treat epilepsy, while today at least 20 FDA-approved medications exist to stop or prevent seizures. Remarkably, my career has spanned the introduction of the concept of the vegetative state and the legalization of brain death.

I have never tired of considering what makes us human, how the brain interprets what our eyes see, or how we can instantly recognize a face not seen for years. I admit that, at times, a sense of mysticism envelops me when contemplating the mystery of human consciousness or the theological question of whether a soul exists separate from the electrical-chemical functioning of the brain.

Early in my education, I was exposed to and fascinated by the writings of Dr. Oliver Sacks. His book, *The Man Who Mistook His Wife for a Hat* (1970), significantly stimulated my interest in neurology. He was a brilliant neurologist and storyteller before he passed away in 2015. He used each patient as an opportunity to explore a human medical predicament. He wrote in a gripping, personal fashion, detailing unusual neurological conditions and their alteration of the victim's functioning. While exploring these maladies scientifically, he wrote with humanity and empathy. His writing was so dramatic that one of his many books, *Awakenings* (1973), about the discovery of Levo-dopa to treat Parkinson's Disease, was made into a movie of the same name.

Dr. Terrance Capistrant, Dr. Richard Foreman, and I started Neurological Associates of St. Paul, P.A. (NASP), the first incorporated neurology specialty practice in the east metro area of the Twin Cities. We began as three clinicians,[1] one nurse, a receptionist, a business office person, an office manager, and a part-time electroencephalography (EEG)[2] technician. In 2015, NASP remained a single specialty private practice neurology group that had grown to 10 physicians supported by a staff of 38 nurses, technicians, and business employees. It had become the largest neurology practice in St. Paul and its suburbs.

> ***"Men ought to know that from the brain, and from the brain only, arise our pleasures, joy, laughter and jests, as well as our sorrows, pains, griefs, and tears."***
> ***—Hippocrates***

The Physician-Patient Contract

Since the beginning of my interest in becoming a doctor, my role as a physician has centered on providing quality patient care according to the ancient physician-patient contract. This contract is spelled out poignantly and clearly in the following modern version of the Hippocratic Oath, as revised in 1964 by Dr. Louis Lasagna, the Academic Dean of Tufts Medical School:

> I swear to fulfill, to the best of my ability and judgment, this covenant: I will respect the hard-won scientific gains of those physicians in whose steps I walk, and gladly share such knowledge as is mine with those who are to follow.
>
> I will apply, for the benefit of the sick, all measures which are required, avoiding those twin traps of overtreatment and therapeutic nihilism.
>
> I will remember that there is art to medicine as well as science, and that warmth, sympathy, and understanding may outweigh the surgeon's knife or the chemist's drug.

---

[1] A clinician is a healthcare professional who diagnoses and treats patients in a hospital, clinic, skilled nursing facility, or in the home. The terms "clinician," "physician," and "doctor" are used interchangeably in this book, and because these professionals are women and men, I will alternate use of the pronouns "he" and "she" interchangeably.

[2] EEG is a noninvasive test that records the electrical activity of the brain.

> I will not be ashamed to say "I know not," nor will I fail to call in my colleagues when the skills of another are needed for a patient's recovery.
>
> I will respect the privacy of my patients, for their problems are not disclosed to me that the world may know. Most especially, must I tread with care in matters of life and death. If it is given to me to save a life, all thanks. But it may also be within my power to take a life; this awesome responsibility must be faced with great humbleness and awareness of my own frailty. Above all, I must not play at God.
>
> I will remember that I do not treat a fever chart, a cancerous growth, but a sick human being, whose illness may affect the person's family and economic stability. My responsibility includes these related problems, if I am to care adequately for the sick.
>
> I will prevent disease whenever I can, for prevention is preferable to cure.
>
> I will remember that I remain a member of society, with special obligations to all my fellow human beings, those sound of mind and body as well as the infirm.
>
> If I do not violate this oath, may I enjoy life and art, respected while I live and remembered with affection thereafter. May I always act so as to preserve the finest traditions of my calling and may I long experience the joy of healing those who seek my help (Lasagna, 1964).

Unfortunately, as I will cover in **Part 1: Healthcare in America**, today's economic "bottom line" is to some extent preempting this physician-patient contract. This might sound like the musing of an aging baby-boomer, reminiscing about the "good old days." Like most physicians, I have strived to practice medicine as the best version of myself, which has not been made easier in 21st century America. The one constant in the world is change, with the field of medicine being no exception. Dramatic advances, progress, and improvements have been achieved, accompanied by an almost obscene increase in expenditures.

Healthcare in America is in crisis. This is in large part due to our system's shift of primary focus from the **patient** to the **process.** To guide a person through life's minor and serious medical maladies humanely today is often subservient to the process of providing medical care. The new norm in medicine places data as the primary concern. This data includes treatment successes and failures, dollars and cents, billing and diagnostic coding, and numbers of patients seen and billed.

Our healthcare system is complex, yet fragmented, while financed by multiple, disparate mechanisms. Despite the enormous costs, regulations, and extensive oversight by the government and insurance companies, our medical outcomes are by multiple measures remarkably mediocre and highly variable.

Minnesota has as mature and well-organized a healthcare system as exists in America. Yet, even in the Twin Cities, anyone who has recently spent significant time in clinics or hospitals is well aware that medicine today is increasingly corporate and less patient-centric. There is a reduced focus on human beings who are anxious, frightened, sick, or dying.

My career has been grounded and enhanced by teaching medicine to students and medical residents. My theories of medical education have become crystallized over the years as has my analysis of the necessary skill set of an effective clinician. These theories of medical education and keys to the practice of medicine are outlined in **Part 2: Becoming a Physician**. I learned these theories and many important life lessons at the bedside.

Early on, I recognized that my patients were providing me an education about life, facing disability and death, and aging. Throughout my career, I conscientiously collected patient quotes and stories, which served as the basis for this book and are highlighted in **Part 3: Life Lessons from My Patients.**

Patients deserve high-quality healthcare that is reasonably priced and accessible. Yet, focusing more intensely on the process rather than the patients has clear unintended consequences. As summarized in **Part 4: What's Next?**, my clarifying these ramifications will hopefully facilitate the necessary alterations of our healthcare system to leverage appropriate improvements without ignoring the key elements of the physician-patient social contract.

While embarking on this writing project, it was my privilege to hear a lecture by Dr. Bennet Omalu, a groundbreaking forensic pathologist who first identified the neurological disease chronic traumatic encephalopathy (CTE) in professional football players. His efforts led to a dramatic battle with the National Football League (NFL), depicted in the movie *Concussion.*

When asked why he vigorously pursued this struggle despite the NFL's attempts to discredit him, he responded:

> We are all one family. What happens to one of us—even the least of us—happens to all of us. As part of that one common family, I think it's a moral duty of mine to share my story like you would share food. To feed the minds, the souls, the hearts and the yearnings of other people. So that if in sharing my story, even if one life is touched, I must have done a lot (Shah, 2016).

Dr. Omalu concluded by saying, "This is your time. This is your stage. There can never be another you in the history of mankind. It is your life to live" (Shah, 2016).

Without knowing me, Dr. Omalu encouraged me to share my story. As he suggests, if the sharing of my story touches even one life, then I will have done my job.

A Migraine In Room 3, A Stroke In Room 4

Part 1

HEALTHCARE IN AMERICA

American healthcare has seen dramatic change. The story of my professional life would be incomplete if not placed in the appropriate context of this change. **Part 1** is an analysis of the American healthcare system and how it has evolved during my career.

The prevailing system is now patterned on a business model with a seemingly endless stream of government regulations and insurance oversight, leading to the erosion of our treatment of patients as individuals. **Chapter 1** identifies six myths that are currently being promoted to inappropriately allay the public's distrust of the evolving system.

Chapter 2 spells out multiple barriers that interfere with the fulfillment of the physician-patient contract. Physician specialization is one way clinicians have found to cope with the rapid advance of medical knowledge and the remarkable stress placed on their personal lives. Unfortunately, the near exponential increase in specialization has unwittingly limited access to care and fostered the burgeoning fragmentation and complexity of care delivery.

Chapter 3 highlights the inefficiencies inherent in this age of subspecialization, which I label "upside down" care.

Despite technological advancements, surgical improvements, and pharmaceutical discoveries, an obligation continues for physicians to educate, counsel, and encourage patients to choose healthy lifestyles. **Chapters 4 and 5** deal with how patients wrestle with embracing healthy choices and comply with prescribed treatment

Chapter One
Myths in the Practice of Medicine Today

"We have no destiny assigned us;
Nothing is certain but the body;
We plan to better ourselves;
The hospitals alone remind us of the equality of man."

—W.H. Auden

Powerful forces have formed today's American healthcare into a complicated, clumsy, fragmented system that is difficult to navigate. Although the core of a quality medical network is the human, intimate relationship between the patient and the physician, our 21st century system is becoming more impersonal, more process-oriented, and less patient-centric.

The goal of each patient encounter should be the treatment of an individual with a problem, placing a person at the center of the system rather than focusing on a medical issue. To enable patients to describe their human condition can be an eye-opening, educational experience. How memorable to hear a patient explain, "My pain feels like a hippopotamus took a bite out of my buttock." Such a relationship not only improves the quality of care, it enhances long-term physician satisfaction that, in turn, minimizes professional burnout.

Patients today desperately need more guidance, education, and communication, not less. Successfully navigating our complex, fragmented system is especially difficult when a person is ill, frightened, or anxious. If the system trends continue unabated, the demand for patient advocates will exponentially increase. I have identified six myths that have been promoted and reinforced by governmental authorities, insurance companies, and provider networks to allay the public's apprehensions and to rationalize the current structure of our healthcare system.

Myth 1: Medical Practitioners Are Interchangeable

Patients in America today are being told that most medical practitioners are interchangeable. Consequently, they are being reassured that, when hospitalized, the doctor who knows them best is not a necessary part of the treatment team. They are told that a hospitalist, typically employed by the hospital, will be competent to provide the best care possible. Hospitalists are doctors typically hired to act as the primary care physician for hospitalized patients, patients without a primary care doctor, or patients whose clinic doctors choose not to assume hospital patient responsibilities.

By necessity, this model requires dramatic emphasis on protocols, published quality measures, and evidence-based medicine. While these are appropriate guidelines in the practice of medicine, wholesale reliance on this generic approach to medicine implies less subjectivity than actually exists in the real world. The best evidence-based medicine must still be applied carefully to unique individuals with inescapable variability that influence the ultimate diagnosis and most appropriate treatment option.

A physician must correctly interpret and document a patient's history before making a diagnosis and treatment plan. Yet, the variable establishment of patient rapport by physicians complicates this process. Different patients will respond to different physicians in various ways. Some patients compound this process by reciting their history in a rambling and disjointed fashion, in an overly detailed way, or in a flamboyant fashion, not knowing what is important and what is not.

Understanding his limited ability to tell his story simply, one patient remarked, "Sorry, doctor, my mouth has no shut-off valve." Another insightful patient who understood her tangential thinking confided in me, "When giving my history, doctor,

I don't always signal my turns." Another worrier described himself as "the President of Ruminators Anonymous."

My nurse often smiled when she suggested that I, at times, functioned as a priest in the office. She came to this conclusion because patients tended to "confess" facts they had withheld from other practitioners or failed to document on impersonal history forms. Patients would admit to having run out of meds without refilling them or to taking less than prescribed.

One epilepsy patient contritely remarked, "I guess one could describe my recent breakthrough seizure as caused by user error." Another patient sheepishly acknowledged that she was actually taking her hated Multiple Sclerosis (MS) shots, prescribed three times per week, "on Sunday, Wednesday, and Sunday."

While all clinicians are trained, each is an individual with a unique combination of strengths and weaknesses. They are not uniformly interchangeable like assembly line workers.

Myth 2: A Clinician Needs No History with a Patient to Provide the Highest Quality of Care

Patients today are being told that no significant disadvantage exists when the evaluating physician has no previous interaction with their needs. When a physician faces a sick patient who is new to him, a conscientiously-obtained detailed history is crucial to formulate an accurate medical assessment. If a physician has no history with a patient, he is indeed handicapped when required to diagnose and establish an effective treatment plan. This is because the quality of the medical assessment will be improved when the active medical issue is placed accurately in appropriate historical context. As the old adage says, "Context matters."

In addition, it is not widely publicized that, as our system depends ever more intensely on physicians with less patient medical history, more testing is ordered. These unnecessary tests increase costs, are wasteful, and can lead to adverse effects. For example, CT scans expose patients to radiation, despite being ordered, at times, as nonchalantly as blood counts. This risk is rarely mentioned by the ordering physician and has only recently begun to be discussed in the lay press.

It is especially troubling when an unnecessary test leads to "red herring" abnormalities that result in unnecessary angst and even more additional testing. Therefore, it is crucial that our system enable and not discourage a patient's established primary care physician to be actively involved whenever her patients need her, especially when the need for hospitalization materializes.

Myth 3: The Physician and Patient Roles Have Not Changed

Patients are being told that their role and their physician's role have not changed. The reality, I believe, is quite different. While our healthcare delivery system has a long history of attempting to be patient-centric, the economics of increasingly corporate-style medicine are becoming the primary focus. The change in focus necessitates a redefinition in the roles of the participants.

The word "patient" comes from the Latin *patiens*, which means "suffering" or "bearing affliction." It does not mean "lives" or "consumer."

The word "doctor" comes from the Latin *docere*, which means "to teach." When physicians are referred to as "providers," this clearly implies a role change. The term "provider" has evolved to incorporate the inclusion in our healthcare system of multiple types of practitioners who have been trained to fulfill, at least in part, a doctor's role. These include nurse practitioners, physician assistants, and nurse clinicians.

The word "provider" does not suggest teacher or professional. Instead, it implies that our clinicians are primarily pre-packaged medical delivery vehicles. Deemphasizing the physician as educator risks minimizing time spent encouraging patients to live healthy lives, to understand their illnesses, and to acquire coping mechanisms.

Throughout this book, I will make the point that the private, human, one-on-one interaction between a doctor and a patient must remain at the core of a healthy system of medical care. Patient-based care must take precedence over the economics of the system. Each individual has a story to tell. While medical encounters can often be quickly and appropriately placed in a neat "diagnostic box," and usually successfully treated by "protocol" by a less trained provider, quality medicine demands more accuracy than "often" or "usually."

A medical history can mimic a detective story, complete with dead ends, "red herrings," unnecessary details, and forgotten or ignored crucial clues or facts. The bedrock of quality medical care is based on identifying the true story, complete with key facts culled from the physician-patient interaction, to which the physician applies his knowledge, experience, and judgment to reach a successful conclusion. This process can be straightforward or significantly complicated.

One patient with a complicated history said it best: "It's not one thing, doctor, it is typically three things." Another elderly patient accurately described his medical condition as "I do not have this, that, or the other thing. I have this, that, and *everything* wrong with me, doc."

When physicians and patients are referred to as providers and customers, role changes are suggested. Our healthcare system should strive to remain patient-centric, while maintaining physicians as diagnosticians and educators.

Myth 4: Physician Extenders Always Provide Reliable Quality Care

Patients are told that alternative medical providers, despite widely varying degrees of education, can function equally and adequately in today's medical world. Patients are told that high-quality care can be provided by physician extenders. This trend is driven to a large extent not by quality of care goals, but by financial incentives to provide less expensive care. In part, the expanding use of physician extenders has also been driven by insufficient numbers of physicians being trained.

Physician extenders are here to stay. They can be efficient and effective, allowing a physician to take responsibility for more patients, while shortening wait times and maintaining quality care. Yet, there must be limitations in their use.

It is no surprise that it is easier to teach a body of facts than it is to teach judgment and the ability to recognize when they "do not know." Nurse practitioners, physician assistants, and other advanced practice nurses must only be used with thoughtful assignments that are consistent with their abilities. Yet, physicians are seldom educated on how to appropriately delegate duties. In addition, physicians are not taught to provide careful oversight.

Over the years, I intermittently tried without much success to employ a nurse practitioner, attempting to relieve my crowded schedule. It was discouraging to be so busy that a patient remarked, "You are like God, Dr. Schanfield. Everyone has heard of you, but no one has ever seen you."

My use of a physician extender was sometimes appreciated by my patients, but often was not. I wished to see my patients and they wished to see me. As one of my MS patients told my nurse practitioner, "Tell Dr. Schanfield that he can run, but he cannot hide."

My son became very ill in a small city in Wisconsin during a summer business internship. He was nauseated, weak, had no appetite, and a fever of 103 degrees. His boss arranged for him to be seen by a medical "provider" at a retail walk-in clinic where an incorrect diagnosis of bilateral ear infection was made, despite my son experiencing no ear pain or hearing loss, and an unnecessary, ineffective antibiotic was prescribed. When he did not improve, he finally agreed to return home where a physician immediately discovered he had mononucleosis with secondary autoimmune, viral hepatitis. He rapidly improved after a short course of steroids. No medical oversight or follow-up had been scheduled by the walk-in clinic and none was ever done.

Many surgeons now use physician extenders to perform routine preoperative and postoperative care. I have indeed been fortunate to share patients with many excellent nurse practitioners in this role, although conscientious oversight is required to assure quality care. By leaving most patient communication to a physician extender, a surgeon risks being perceived as primarily concerned with technical surgical issues rather than the patients themselves.

For many reasons, physician extenders are here to stay, but must be educated, utilized, and overseen appropriately and consistently.

Myth 5: Technology Compensates for Fragmentation of Care

Patients in America are told that technology will improve medical care in many ways. The electronic medical record (EMR) has been an amazing technological advancement. The dramatic and relatively rapid switch to the EMR required leadership and vision. President Obama led the way. As reviewed by Timothy Johnson and Julia Marcotte, "When President-elect Barack Obama took office in 2009, one of his first commitments was that within five years, all American citizens' medical records would be computerized." The primary motivation for this change was provided by "the Centers of Medicare and Medicaid Services' commitment to make incentive payments to hospitals and providers, along with a penalty for failure to adopt electronic health records" (Johnson & Marcotte, 2016, pp. 34-36).

Patients are reassured that the EMR provides immediate access to all necessary information for physicians unfamiliar with a patient, allowing them to always provide the highest level of care. Patients are guaranteed that the EMR will compensate for their being treated by less well-trained practitioners. Patients are told that the EMR will compensate for the fragmentation of care, even allowing more patients to be seen in less time.

To work, our system must remain centered on the patient-physician interaction. The EMR must be used to improve patient outcomes, while increasing—not decreasing—the physician time directly spent with the patient.

Until this new electronic age of medicine, documentation of medical care had taken a backseat. A disconnect has existed for decades when comparing a physician's skill of observation and medical decision-making with the ability to accurately record and measure their thought processes (Goldenberg, 2016). It turns out that huge amounts of data are generated by the clinical practice of medicine, which makes it "difficult to determine the most meaningful data to collect." The physician-patient interaction certainly contains important data to be obtained and documented, however, this can be over-emphasized. As famously stated by sociologist William Bruce Cameron, "Not everything that counts can be counted, and not everything that can be counted counts" (Cameron, 1963).

The transition to the new electronic era of medicine has been difficult. It appears as though the unintended consequences to patient care were never seriously considered. The EMR is currently widely viewed as a barrier separating the patient from the doctor. As one patient put it to me, "You don't have to apologize for focusing on the computer so much of the time, doctor. All patients are getting used to seeing their doctor in profile."

The EMR is here to stay and promises significant advantages, despite numerous faults, escalating costs, unintended consequences, and unfulfilled lofty expectations.[3] Unfortunately, many of the EMR systems were rushed to market before they were perfected. Every few months, new and updated versions are instituted, taking additional physician time to master.

It appears that the EMRs are largely constructed by software engineers who seem to lack knowledge of the intricacies and nuances of the practice of medicine. Many of the systems in practice are cumbersome, expensive, malfunction at unpredictable times, and are "not well-matched to clinical workflow" patterns of physicians, leading to "clinicians' frustrations and objections" (Goldenberg, 2016, pp. 81-86).

It seems clear that the EMR is no longer a thing of the future. Today's computer programs can analyze a lot of data in the patient health record. Computers can be programmed to alert the practitioner to possible allergic reactions, suggest possible treatment and testing protocols, or recommend follow-up appointments. However, these systems don't possess common sense. Some of these systems have so many notifications and alerts as to trigger "alert fatigue."

A 2016 study calculated that each primary care physician surveyed in Texas received an average of 77 notifications per day. Specialists fared better, averaging only 29 notifications per day (Murphy et. al, 2016). I don't mean to imply that physicians did not receive dozens of messages in the pre-EMR era, but the messages were often sent by knowledgeable nurses and secretaries, who enhanced the messages with their judgment and common sense.

In the past, chart documentation was primarily accomplished by dictation and transcribed by knowledgeable professionals who could improve the dictations, saving physicians time. The transcriptionists are gone. Now the physician typically types directly into the record, fills in the blanks in rigid, prefab outlines, or uses voice recognition software.

The voice recognition technology is rapidly becoming widespread. This "dragon" software types directly into the medical record what it assumes the physician said. In theory, voice recognition should allow a physician to efficiently and accurately

---

[3] An article published by the *Boston Business Journal* states that The RAND Corporation, whose "optimism for EMR in 2005 helped initiate a government and industry push for their adoption," walked back their claims. "RAND originally predicted widespread use of the EMR could save the U.S. healthcare system at least $81 billion a year. RAND now says that figure was overstated." The report came about after studies "found little savings at hospitals from health IT adoption." (Moore, 2013)

populate the medical record. However, these systems were also rushed to market before being ready for prime time, thus requiring careful proofreading, which physicians rarely have the time or the energy to do.

Reminiscent of the age of illegible physician handwriting, some of these records are uninterpretable and riddled with computer-generated errors. The following are examples of computer-generated voice recognition transcription errors:

- "The man had genital deafness in the left ear." (Should be "congenital.")
- "His memory was fine until his ovaries stopped working." (Should be "kidneys.")
- "This letter should be sent to: Arthritis and Rheumatology Consultants in the Vagina." (Should be "in Edina," a city in Minnesota.)
- "There was a Ms. Interpretation of the pathology report." (Should be "misinterpretation.")
- "The patient was in R offices on May 1." (Should be "our.")
- "We discussed who she would C next after my retirement." (Should be "see.")
- "A Mr. Angela Graham will be scheduled." (Should be an "MR Angiogram.")
- "His eye was shocked." (Should be "shut.")
- "Pursley[4] reviewed the records." (Should be "personally.")
- "The testes came back normal." (Should be "tests.")
- The patient was prepped for surgery and raped in the usual manner." (Should be "draped.")

One day in the hospital, my medical student was proofreading my hospital voice recognition patient visit note. She caught an error and urged me to repeat what I dictated until the computer software got it right. I was trying to dictate that "the patient had a right-sided hemiplegia."[5] The computer initially typed "him my plegia." I repeated the phrase and the computer typed "MI plegia." Following the third try, the computer typed "hemiparesis."[6] After my fourth try, the computer typed "hemiparesis plegia." Following my fifth attempt, the computer typed "him on a plegia." The computer correctly typed "hemiplegia" after my sixth try. Success was finally achieved!

---

[4] Pursley or *Portulaca oleracea* is a trailing plant native to Eurasia.

[5] Hemiplegia is a medical term for a complete paralysis of one side of the body.

[6] Hemiparesis is a medical term for weakness on one side of the body, though not complete paralysis.

Unlike the physician's staff, the EMR has only data and is unable to seamlessly "exchange and integrate patient health information" (Johnson & Marcotte, 2016, p. 34). A 2016 study by Dr. Christine Sinsky "found that primary care physicians were spending 38 hours a month after hours doing data entry work; in other words, working a full extra week every month doing documentation once their clinics had closed, between 7:00 p.m. and 7:00 a.m." (Clark, 2016a). This was coupled with data showing that physicians spent 44% of their day doing data entry work and 28% of the day with patients. The article highlights ten ways EMRs contribute to inefficient physician work and "what some doctors have started to call EHR[7] pajama time," included below:

1. Too many clicks: Clearly the builders of the software do not use the system.
2. Note bloat: Many pages of duplicated facts with little highlight of conclusions.
3. Poor workflow: The EMR workflow does not match how clinicians work or think.
4. Lack of focus on the patient.
5. No support for team care: Each caregiver's notes are prepared separately, after separate log-ins.
6. Distracted hikes to the printer: The printer is rarely in the patient room.
7. Single-use workstations so physicians and nurses cannot work side-by-side.
8. Small monitors making it unusual to view a lot of information simultaneously.
9. Long sign-in process: Confidentiality and safety trump physician ease of use and time expenditure.
10. Underuse of students as scribes[8]: A UCLA study found these assistants save three hours per day of physician time. (Clark, 2016a)

Today's evolving systems of medical documentation and oversight have the unintended consequence of isolating physicians by demanding a larger share of the physician workday be spent away from the bedside. The physician's staff is less able to share the physician's workload of medical documentation that is demanded by today's healthcare system. Our medical system now stipulates a detailed and cogent delineation of the physician's thought process. This process is more complex than it appears, however, involving a vast array of information and judgment not easily documented.

---

[7] Sometimes the EMR is referred to as an electronic health record (EHR).

[8] Scribes are typically students who are included in the physician-patient interaction and are hired to enter physician notes into the EMR.

To be clear, medicine is not the only profession to have increased reliance on technology. Dr. Sherry Turkle, an MIT professor of social studies of science and tech nology, has written extensively on the dehumanizing influence of technology today (Dominick, 2017). Her book titles include *Reclaiming Conversation: The Power of Talk in the Digital Age* and *Alone Together: Why We Expect More from Technology and Less from Each Other.*

Certainly, most physicians would agree with Dr. Turkle's assertions that conversation is the most humanizing thing we do, while we are doing less of it these days. She stresses that "a flight from conversation undermines our relationships, creativity, and productivity" and that "reclaiming face-to-face conversation can help us regain lost ground." She clarifies the difference between our always being connected in a technological universe and meaningful face-to-face conversation (Dominick, 2017).

The difficulty sharing patient information between EMRs, the prevalent alert fatigue, the dramatic cost of these systems, the mismatch of the electronic data collection systems to efficient and quality clinical medicine's workflow patterns, and the interference with meaningful patient-physician dialogue are major challenges that must be overcome to experience the full potential of the institution of the EMR. We will get there, but have a long way to go.

Myth 6: Protocols and Checklists Assure Quality Care

Patients in America are told that a regimented, protocol-driven approach to medicine will prevent malpractice. It is indeed appropriate to continue to search for ways to avoid mistakes. It is indeed appropriate to use protocols.

Although memorizing lists, protocols, statistics, anatomy diagrams, chemical formulas, physiological systems, and drugs is certainly the backbone of best medical practice, it is actually the easy part. The key to practicing high-quality medicine and avoiding mistakes is found in the additional years of concerted work, study, and experience needed to create a highly skilled diagnostician who can apply the data, protocols, and facts to an individual person. Every patient is unique, with her own medical history, health needs, goals, and wishes.

It is useful to have "cookbook" protocols readily available for today's hassled and hurried clinician. However, just as the use of a cookbook does not guarantee the success of the chef, so it is in its use in medicine. Like cooking, medicine is in part an art that needs to be "practiced."

No role exists, in my opinion, for a cookbook approach to medicine that does not stress the art of applying the facts to a unique individual in a specific circumstance. To be effective, the application of the protocols must match the needs of each individual patient, which can be unpredictable and, at times, difficult to ascertain. For instance, one of our standard memory assessment protocols asks for the patient to spell the word "world" backwards. One of my patients stood up and began to walk backwards in the exam room while spelling "w-o-r-l-d."

In reality, the patient visit may not be about the patient's initial chief complaint at all. This fact can lead to miscommunication and confusion when the evaluation process centers on the rapid pigeonholing of the patient's issues with rigid forms and protocols.

Prematurely invoking a protocol risks leading the patient evaluation in the wrong direction. In addition, relying on protocols tends to limit the free-flowing interaction between the patient and physician. This in turn decreases the number of memorable interactions and further leads to the impersonalization of medicine. Rigid lines of questioning allow the physician less opportunity to invoke a patient's insightful observations and less chance that the patient's emotional state will be revealed.

Complicated communication with patients can lead to the failure of forms, protocols, and computerized checklists. The medical answers may not be "black or white." Where does the patient write in a checklist, "I have a host of horribles"? Our form was obviously inappropriate for a man who filled in the blanks, "Married: Yes; Spouse: One." Where in a computerized protocol will an elderly man, who turned out to have Alzheimer's Disease, rationalize his memory issues by saying, "They don't pay me to think anymore, so I don't."

Successful use of protocols and checklists occurs when they are used as screening tools to begin the patient-physician conversation, rather than to replace physician-patient interactions. The key to effective utilization of protocols and cookbook diagnostic and treatment regimens is their ability to aid in the avoidance of mistakes, not their ability to replace physician judgment and experience.

Summary

Six myths have been propagated to allay our fears about the dramatic changes taking place in American medicine in the 21st century. Once spelled out in black and white, the shortcomings in these proclamations are obvious. Few would admit that all medical practitioners are created equal or that a clinician with less patient history is not disadvantaged. By referring to patients as "lives" or "consumers" and physicians as "providers," a cataclysmic change in the roles of patients and physicians is suggested. Although physician extenders certainly are important, to be successful, their roles must be thoughtfully delineated and delegated while meticulous oversight is maintained.

Anyone who has recently been a patient has experienced the EMR interfering with the intimacy of the physician visit. The EMR must improve and clear significant hurdles to live up to its lofty expectations and still foster an appropriate level of intimacy during a physician visit.

Finally, while protocols and checklists have an appropriate role in medicine today, they are obviously useless and potentially harmful if used by clinicians devoid of judgement and wisdom, the fundamental keys to the successful practice of medicine.

One of my partners, Dr. Zohreh Mahdavi, said it best: "When all is said and done with EMR, protocols, testing, quality audits, and computerized information sources, it is still best for a doctor to listen and to think."

Chapter 2
Barriers to Fulfilling the Physician-Patient Contract

On the long and complex path to provide the best bedside and clinic care possible, today's physicians find that the current healthcare system has placed multiple barriers in their way. These barriers interfere with clinicians' ability to provide individualistic, humane, and up-to-date care for their patients. The American system is in transition.

While the art of medicine has forever been a work in progress, never have as many external demands been placed on physicians. These powerful forces are demanding uniformity, quality, accountability, increased productivity at a decreased cost, and compulsively detailed documentation. The changes in healthcare involve delivery, documentation, insurance, reimbursement, pharmaceutical preauthorization, government regulation, and oversight.

While some of these demands are reasonable and should improve care, others are not. Unfortunately, many of these forces, even when seemingly appropriate, are requiring rapid changes in our system, which have had significant and, at times, unfortunate unintended consequences. These unintended consequences, in my opinion, have led to the erection of nine barriers between the patient and the physician.

1. Less Physician Time Devoted to Direct Patient Care

As change has accelerated, the physician today finds that, each week, more time is devoted to acquiring and mastering new skill sets that have little to do with patient care. Rather, these skills involve documentation, coding, and billing. The resulting decrease in direct contact between the physician and the patient, while an inappropriate goal, is the new reality. Clinicians must decide to spend the majority of their time practicing medicine with face-to-face time with the patient sacredly guarded. Doing so should diminish patient distrust and increase the satisfaction of patients and physicians alike.

It is a fact that clinic visits are short, difficult to schedule, and filled with paperwork and questionnaires. However, adequate time must be available for the physician to make sure the patient and family understand the diagnosis, the plan, the likely prognosis, and the next steps. The physician and his staff are responsible for establishing the clinic schedules, which need to allow adequate time for educating the patient and family. This includes explaining specific diagnostic steps and treatment options that may include lifestyle changes.

The aging of our population compounds the needs and complexity of typical clinic visits. As one 85-year-old gentleman remarked, "I'm not old, but I was around when Moby Dick was a minnow and Christ was a corporal."

2. Transition to Large, Corporate Physician Groups

For much of the last 50 years, most physicians were largely self-employed in partnerships or small professional associations. As a matter of fact, when the Mayo Clinic evolved into a group practice model with physicians' salaries set by the Clinic, it was accused of illegal fee splitting, because the fees were shared among the practitioners, not strictly given to the physician who did the work.

By the second decade of the 21st century, physicians are commonly employed in very large groups. As of 2016, "fewer than 20 percent of doctors are in solo practice" (Scheffler & Glied, 2016). These large groups are now typically run by non-physician administrators. This change has led to the eroding of physician responsibility and loyalty to their medical practices. With no ownership and limited control over their professional lives, a dramatic increase in workplace physician mobility has taken place.

Not surprisingly, patients recognize and suffer from the lack of a long-term commitment by physicians, resulting in increased disruption of the physician-patient social contract. The lack of a stable physician workforce is a significant drawback to medical care in America today. It leads directly to fragmented medical care and increased medical expenditures.

It is not surprising that a large percentage of patients have trouble naming their primary care provider and express significant dissatisfaction with our system. I typically ask my patients who their family doctor or internist is. One patient responded, "Google." It is clear that patients are feeling more like numbers as part of a profit/loss equation rather than human beings with problems.

Less permanent patient-physician relationships lead to quality of care concerns and increased expenditures. The musical chairs phenomenon of providing medical care leads to inappropriate diagnostic and treatment plans. It has long been a bedrock assumption in medicine that, to get the best medical history from a patient, a doctor should have a history with the patient. The most successful physicians apply medical "best practice parameters" to the specific needs of an individual patient. Unfortunately, the less a physician knows about the patient, the more difficult the task of identifying the patient's specific needs.

> ***"When at last we are sure, you've been properly pilled. Then a few paper forms, must be properly filled. So that you and your heirs may be properly billed."***
> ***—Dr. Seuss***

Every patient is unique with a distinct medical history and specific health needs, goals, and wishes. Unfortunately, in the business model of medicine, the appreciation of the skill of treating a unique individual in a specific circumstance is minimized. This is in large part due to the difficulty in objectively identifying how successful a physician is in acquiring this skill set. Therefore, today's large group practices tend to focus on measures of productivity, such as patient encounters, billings, and test orders, while assuming that malpractice threats will assure quality care.

In recognition of this new reality of unhappiness of the providers and the patients, the hospital and clinic networks are measuring patient satisfaction. Unfortunately, adding more paperwork to a patient's clinic visit or hospital stay is not being met with enthusiasm, nor is it revealing new and useful information. Everywhere in corporate America, we are being asked to waste time filling out satisfaction questionnaires. This "going through the motions" neither advances patient loyalty nor respect. It is obvious what the problems are and more paperwork is not the answer.

3. Fragmentation of Medical Care

Significant fragmentation of healthcare currently exists both in the clinics and in the hospitals. This has come about as an unintended consequence of the dramatic forces of change occurring today. One exasperated patient, who lived alone, asked, "How am I going to get to the newly-ordered physical therapy, since I was also instructed not to drive?" Another patient was reassured that home care, which he was instructed to set up, would allow for his quick hospital discharge. However, with no coordination between the hospital and the home care services, his recovery was threatened when he was unable to get a home visit for three weeks.

Clinic Care: Remarkably, in the last decade, most primary care clinic doctors have chosen not to follow and care for their clinic patients when admitted to the hospital. This dramatic change in practice patterns has been driven in part by rapidly changing and ever expanding medical advancements of diagnoses and treatment in the hospitals. It is not easy to keep abreast and be current with both hospital and clinic medicine.

To a large degree, however, the clinic physicians have relinquished their hospital responsibilities because of lifestyle choices and significant government and insurance influences. These influences have dramatically increased the cost and overhead of running medical clinics in the 21st century.

Complex insurance company billing requirements must be dealt with in exacting detail. Electronic medical records, with frequent upgrades and breakdowns, are extremely expensive to purchase and maintain. At each clinic visit, patients are reminded about concealed weapons regulations and insurance copays. They are required to show photo identification and proof of insurance, and then asked to fill out multiple, onerous forms and questionnaires. Only then will the patient see the physician, or possibly a "physician extender," such as a nurse practitioner, for a few minutes.

An elderly clinic patient, believing that her driver's license picture was ugly, refused to show it to her primary care physician's new, young receptionist saying, "Go ask the doctor who I am. I have seen him for 15 years! I don't know who you are."

The most direct way to cover the ever-increasing overhead costs of running a clinic has been to have each clinician spend as much time as possible seeing patients. In other words, physicians have significant financial inducements to see more clinic patients. It is much less efficient for a clinic doctor to regularly schedule time to attend to hospitalized patients as the hospital patient census cannot be known from day-to-day.

With little financial incentive to evaluate and console sick hospital patients, and ever increasing clinic pressures to see more outpatients, today's typical primary care physician spends all day in the clinic or in the hospital. In the light of these changes, the patient's needs are no longer of paramount concern.

Once the system placed such a high value on the economics of healthcare, the physician became responsible to see a specific number of patients per day, without regard to patient needs. In 2016, Paul Berrisford was the COO of Entira Family Clinics, a St. Paul-based physician owned and run group of clinics. He described the current system as "the crazy, volume-based hamster wheel medical system that pays doctors by how many office visits they squeeze in each day" (Olson, 2016).

Berrisford went on to lament that his clinics cannot bill for their care managers, nurses, pharmacists, and therapists. These trained individuals counsel chronically ill patients to adopt healthier lifestyles, increase their medication compliance, and guide them through the fragmented system of care. Clinics such as his "have to take on these costs that will lower the cost of healthcare, with no possible way to bill for them" (Olson, 2016).

As medication and testing expenses increase, it has become common for insurance companies to refuse payment for medications and procedures. They require the patient and the clinic go through additional hoops of reporting information, despite currently being accessible electronically.

These hoops entail additional physician dictations or telephone conversations, adding many more hours of clinic nursing or physician time spent away from the patient. I presume this process is calculated to decrease, or at least delay, insurance payments, although it is often touted as being a quality of care safeguard.

Sadly, an MS patient of mine experienced a disease flare-up when she ran out of medication because her insurance company suddenly refused to pay for the expensive prescription refill until more information was submitted. She could not afford to pay for the drug until the insurance payment was reinstituted. No quality of care issue was apparent as the medication was controlling her disease and was "standard of care," according to the American Academy of Neurology.

Further increasing the cost and complexity of clinic medicine today is governmental oversight. Unfortunately, the "modest" financial benefits of treating a Medicare patient, which when combined with Medicare's "systematic undervaluing of care provision, is threatening the long-term participation of the neurologist in the program" (Dorsey, 2016, p. 11). This is compounded by the fact that "approximately 80% of Medicare patients have at least one chronic condition, and yet have trouble accessing appropriate care" (Dorsey, 2016, p. 11).

Remarkably, a 2011 study documented that 42% of Parkinson patients don't see a neurologist. Denied the benefit of specialized care, these patients are 20% more likely to fracture a hip, be placed in a nursing home, or die. "While distance and disability likely contribute to the access problem, financial incentives that continue to favor institutions over patients are likely to be a major contributing factor" (Dorsey, 2016, p. 11).

Because of the unstable physician workforce often requiring new health clinicians, increased patient mobility, and frequent insurance coverage changes, patients are now more than ever dealing with new practitioners. Besides struggling to understand a new patient's medical and social issues, clinic physicians are also pressured to focus on documentation, billing, and coding.

On October 1, 2015, the tenth version of diagnostic coding was introduced. It includes approximately 68,000 new outpatient codes and another 68,000 codes for hospital and surgical procedures. Can there really be that many different diagnoses?

Separate codes exist for a right carpal tunnel surgery and a left carpal tunnel surgery. One code covers an alligator bite and a different code a crocodile bite. After a patient heard me complain about this complexity, she commented, "Dr. Schanfield, you should be happy. There are actually 23 species of crocodilians."

Amazingly, a code exists for "being sucked into a jet engine." Remember the Dos Equis commercials featuring the "most interesting man in the world"? In November of 2015, I received a text with the picture of the most interesting man in the world remarking, "I don't always get sucked into a jet engine, but when I do, I use ICD-10:

V97.33XD" (Drummond, n.d.).

In January 2016, I attempted to count the number of codes for a patient with an ischemic stroke (caused by a clot) with or without complications. I came up with an incredible 326 different stroke codes, excluding TIA (a stroke syndrome which clears completely) and intracranial hemorrhage (a stroke caused by a ruptured blood vessel rather than a clot within the vessel) (Schoenberg, 2016).

As more physician time is spent on government and insurance documentation, coding, and billing tasks, both physician and patient dissatisfaction has grown. This dissatisfaction has further diminished patient and physician loyalty, while fragmenting care.

Hospital Care: A new medical specialist, called a "hospitalist," has emerged in the 21st century. As I mentioned in **Chapter 1**, hospitalists are doctors typically hired to act as the primary care physician for hospitalized patients, patients without a primary care doctor, or patients whose clinic doctors choose not to assume hospital responsibilities. They are typically employed by the hospital as shift workers. With the focus on the process and the providers rather than the patient, even a readmitted patient is rarely seen by the same physician.

Who would have imagined that, when a person became ill and in need of hospitalization, her doctor would rarely be at the bedside? When patients were managed primarily by private practice physicians from the clinic, continuity of care and the patient's welfare were paramount, as it should be.

As never before, the hospitalist must answer directly to the institution that pays his salary when questions arise. Some of these questions are predictably quality of care related, although some are associated with the patient's length of stay and the amount of testing performed.

The hospitalist is paid to provide good care, complete all the mandated paperwork required, and manage the length of the hospital stay, including estimating the discharge date upon admission. She then organizes the discharge and follow-up plans with other providers, including nursing home or rehab transfers if the patient cannot return home directly.

Some hospitalists receive bonuses if patients are discharged more quickly than expected, especially early in the day. To try to discourage short and inappropriate admissions, Medicare now requires that the treating hospital physician guarantee upon admission that the patient requires hospitalization that will span at least two midnights. In addition, Medicare typically refuses to pay for a subsequent nursing home stay after a hospitalization of less than three days duration.

This new hospitalist specialty comes with concerns that are beginning to be discussed in the medical literature. In response to some of these issues, the hospitalists in one Springfield, Oregon, hospital have formed a union (Fallik, 2016a). Significant pressures are being imposed on these clinicians to see additional patients, discharge patients in a more timely manner, and increase the numbers of hours worked. The Oregon physicians felt these pressures were "compromising the quality of patient care" (Fallik, 2016a, p. 28). The hospitalists identified "ominous trends in how the quality of their work is measured and valued" (Fallik, 2016a, p. 33). Time will tell if physician unions become the norm in America.

Many physicians feel that they have lost control and, indeed, many medical centers "have seen a massive expansion in administrative hierarchy over the last two decades. The administration includes both doctors and business people, including some from outside management companies, who are far removed from the front lines of the ward and clinics, but nonetheless dictate what they believe is the best way for patient care to occur" (Fallik, 2016a, p. 33).

Dr. Joshua P. Klein, chair of the American Academy of Neurology Neurohospitalist Section, observed that these dictated changes "often prove to be ill-conceived" as they are propagated to require physicians to take care of more and sicker patients most cheaply. Dr. Klein lamented:

> As these initiatives are rolled out, clinicians are typically first incentivized toward compliance, but later penalized for failure to maintain compliance. If an initiative ultimately fails, as many have, there never seems to be accountability on the part of the administrators for all the clinicians' time and resources wasted, let alone that the initiative had any positive effect on patient care in the first place" (Fallik, 2016a, p. 33).

The hospitalists are typically intelligent and capable, but rarely have a history with the patient. Despite increasing hospital oversight and emphasis on quality of care measures, part of the escalating hospital costs are undoubtedly due to hospitalists' lack of familiarity with the patients.

Many serious issues need addressing. It's astonishing that less than 40% of discharged hospital patients today can name their hospital attending physician. In one survey, two-thirds of the patients were discharged without knowing their diagnosis (Joshi, 2015). The patients are often elderly with multiple maladies and issues. One patient later told me that she had a complication after discharge, yet she did not know which physician to call.

Hospital experiences can be difficult, exhausting, and confusing. An elderly, hospitalized man, who was repeatedly asked orientation questions such as his name, date, and location, finally cried out to me, "I must be here incognito. No one seems to know who I am."

I experienced first-hand fragmentation of care in the hospital, when hospitalized overnight for a minor ailment. Even though the hospital staff wanted to treat me as a V.I.P., I suffered an exhausting night. A nursing assistant woke me at 5:00 a.m. to take my temperature. A different assistant returned at 5:30 a.m. to take my pulse and blood pressure. The phlebotomist[9] woke me at 6:00 a.m. to draw blood for routine morning labs. At 6:30 a.m., yet another person had me stand to record my weight. At 7:00 a.m., a nurse, whom I knew well, arrived for her day shift and came into my room to greet me. I was exhausted and crabby, but I doubt that she understood why I was unhappy to see her just then.

As I experienced firsthand, many people do not find the hospital a restful place to be sick, let alone to begin recuperating. On my rounds one morning, I attempted to interview a patient who was eating breakfast. Unhappy with yet another interruption, who could blame him when he remarked, "Come back later, doctor, I am sleeping"?

4. Issues Concerning Quality of Care

Improving quality care is of crucial importance and dramatically relevant. I participated in a quality of care webinar sponsored by the National Quality Forum (NQF) that reported a startling statistic: In 35 million hospital admissions, 100,000 deaths, and 1,000,000 serious medical adverse events occurred. Contrast these actual results with a Six Sigma statistical prediction that an acceptable number of adverse medical errors should have been 1,105 (Grau, 2016).

[9] Phlebotomist is a person who draws blood for laboratory tests.

Because of the failure of the American system to routinely deliver superior outcomes despite enormous expenditures, evaluating quality of care is now being more seriously addressed. This has led to inordinately complex—and questionably appropriate—documentation procedures. Healthcare delivery is complicated and measuring it can indeed be a labyrinthine task.

A rush to address quality measures has, at times, led to poorly thought-out reporting measures. The need to fulfill these new and required parameters unfortunately interrupts the intimate, human interaction of the patient visit, often leaving little time for other important issues to be tabulated. The first version of government mandated "meaningful use" was abandoned in 2016 after a couple of years of disruptive and poorly conceived implementation.

5. Increasing Specialization and Subspecialization in Medicine

It has taken me a number of years to realize that the dramatic expansion of subspecialty training programs and the significantly increased numbers of subspecialists in medicine are barriers to the physician-patient social contract. Rarely does an internal medicine resident go into practice without first taking a subspecialty fellowship.

Even in the specialties, a dramatic emphasis on further fellowship training has occurred. In my own field for example, most neurology residents spend another one to three years getting further training in sleep, Parkinson's Disease, stroke, headache, peripheral nerve disorders, dementia, epilepsy, or brain tumors. The justifications are obvious, but so are the limitations and disruptions of care. The further a physician is from the primary care of a patient, the more the patient becomes a "problem" rather than a "person with a problem." This leads to additional fragmentation of care.

6. Physician Compensation Favoring Surgery and Procedures over Patient Care

For decades, the medical reimbursement system in America has favored "doing something" as opposed to talking with, counseling, or educating people. According to Dr. Douglas Wood, Medical Director of the Center for Innovation at the Mayo Clinic, America's healthcare system "is tied to an outdated, traditional medical model" (Wood, 2016, p. 14).

The existing structure is entrenched, and we find our country, for the most part, still burdened with skyrocketing pharmaceutical prices, shackled to reimbursement systems based on sickness care, and wrestling with rising insurance costs, despite the Affordable Care Act (Wood, 2016, p. 14).

Dr. Wood opines that the Affordable Care Act significantly reduces the number of Americans without access to medical care, but does little to improve its affordability.

Surgical procedures are more highly reimbursed than examining and talking with patients, even if the same amount of time and energy are expended. With the financial incentive favoring surgery, many surgeons spend little time beforehand discussing the surgery and sometimes even less time postoperatively with the patients. Some of my patients have never seen the surgeon postoperatively!

One of my retired partners underwent a complicated multi-level spinal fusion at a renowned multi-specialty center. While he did see the surgeon postoperatively, the cursory visits never included a neurological examination. While efficient, this was not an example of quality follow-up care.

Primary care and pediatrics have traditionally been compensated the least. Historically, this has been balanced by the reward of meaningful patient-physician interactions, with time well spent in communication and counseling patients and families. A wonderful pediatrician I know well has described himself as "a psychiatrist who also looks in ears."

However, as the financial and documentation burdens increase, and the compensation diminishes, a point occurs where the system loses its mainstay and backbone of care: the primary care physician. This further leads to fragmentation of care.

Dr. Leana Wen, the Commissioner of the Baltimore City Health Department and co-author of *When Doctors Don't Listen: How to Avoid Misdiagnoses and Unnecessary Tests*, was asked, "If you could change or eliminate something about the healthcare system, what would it be?" She responded just as I would:

> Financial incentives. Our financial incentives are completely skewed in the wrong direction. . . . I would change our entire reimbursement system so that we're paying for things we do **for** patients rather than for things that we're doing **to** them. I would change our incentive structure so that our primary care fields are reimbursed the highest (Firth, 2016b).

I must admit, however, that many patients actually demand "action, tests, and treatments," while discounting the value of time spent in communication and counseling with their physician. I have too often heard the phrase, "the doctor did nothing for me," when no testing or interventions were recommended, even when the doctor appropriately avoided ordering the unnecessary interventions.

7. Escalation of Healthcare Costs

Many reasons exist for the continuing and, at times, dramatic increases in costs, including:

- Well-publicized and exciting new medical advances, such as advanced and effective diagnostic and treatment options, including new implants and surgical procedures.
- Unstable physician workforce, which leads directly to fragmented medical care, increased medical expenditures, and inefficient care.
- Remarkable increases in technology expenditures unrelated to delivering care, highlighted by the EMR.
- Dramatic increases in prices, including well-publicized, out-of-control pharmaceutical prices.
- Ever-expanding patient demand for more testing and treatment.
- Growing overhead clinic costs.
- Perverse physician incentives to "do something."
- Physician time saved by ordering tests rather than convincing patients they are unnecessary.
- Costs of measuring medical expenditures, which "has created a multi-billion dollar measurement industry that has lost sight of the need to improve health" (Wood, 2016, p. 15).
- Aging of the population.

It remains common, unfortunately, for patients and their families not to have clearly established how much treatment an elderly relative would want when a crisis occurs. It is well known that a large percentage of a person's medical expenditures occur in the last few months of life with little benefit achieved.

An all-too-common scenario is often played out in the treatment of end-stage cancer patients. Some oncologists have reputations of ordering a new chemotherapy treatment rather than having an honest, although likely protracted and uncomfortable, conversation with the patient and family about imminent death. I saw this firsthand at my father's last oncology visit a few brief days before he died.

I have briefly mentioned above and detailed in **Chapter 1** the dramatic costs of the electronic medical record (EMR). The systems are expensive to buy, maintain, and master. The promise that once these systems became universal they would avoid duplication of testing, save time, and save billions of dollars has proved impossible to deliver and probably was unrealistic and unattainable.

With a wide variety of systems in use, it can be cumbersome for them to "talk" to each other, so that it is still often quicker and easier for the doctor to repeat a test, such as a CT scan, rather than find the previous result.

Hidden from the public is the fact that the EMR facilitates medical providers to "upshift" billing codes, another reason for escalating costs. The systems allow clinicians to easily "pull" information from previous patient encounters into a current visit, justifying a more expensive billing code. Not uncommonly, the record rapidly becomes bloated by these billing code justifications, at times obscuring the key and pertinent facts pertaining to the patient encounter.

8. Changes in Patient Population

With the economization of physician networks, it is not surprising that patients' opinions of doctors and their experiences at the office are changing. Unfortunately, it is becoming common to hear, "I love you, doctor. I just don't have much faith in you guys these days." It is not lost on the patients that their long-standing social contract with physicians has changed. It is not lost on them that the contract now seems to be based on economics first with patient needs second.

In this age of abundant news, we are bombarded with medical information, which is at times useful, at times misleading, and at times incorrect. This tends to raise patients' expectations. Unfortunately, increased patient expectations are not often coupled with the knowledge that health starts with patients taking responsibility as active members of the treatment team. Today's patients often want to be "fixed" quickly with little effort on their part. "Doc," asserted one of my patients, "you get me to 100 years old, and I'll take it the rest of the way."

Yet, a quality physician must attempt to impart to her patients a sense of individual responsibility, while not raising the person's ire. Indeed, not enough emphasis is made of the fact that a correct diagnosis that will hopefully lead to successful treatment typically starts with the patient accurately conveying the medical history. Patients should be educated to:

- Think through in advance what will likely occur at the doctor's office.
- Bring up important issues early in a doctor visit instead of saving important revelations or key questions for when the physician stands to leave.
- Know the dosages of their medications and what has been tried in the past.
- Be accompanied by family members or friends who can help fill in their medical history and important family history details.
- Be truthful in addition to being prepared.
- Accept responsibility to carry out the treatment plan.
- Speak up if they do not understand a diagnosis or proposed course of treatment.

In his article, "Misdiagnosis Solutions Generated by St. Paul Think Tank," Jeremy Olson assigns responsibility to patients to communicate eight characteristics of their symptoms to their doctor: "quantity, quality, aggravating factors, alleviating factors, setting, associated symptoms, location, timing" (2015).

I was once convinced that a woman had typical migraine headaches until she clarified her complaints by saying, "On second thought, I don't really have headaches. My head feels out of order." Another patient, who turned out to have had a small stroke, complained, "My speech has developed a hitch in my giddy-up."

When patients understand and are actively engaged in their own health, the system works best. Consequently, doctors should take time to educate their patients as to their importance in the process (Hawton, 2016). Yet, educating patients can be difficult. It was not easy to educate a man who said to me, "I can't hear you doctor, because I don't have my hearing aids," to which his daughter responded, "Dad, you don't have hearing aids."

9. Changes in Physician Employment

> *"Cure sometimes, treat often, comfort always."*
> *—Hippocrates*

Characteristics of the typical physician job description are changing, triggering increasing dissatisfaction with the profession. After years of long hours and increasing family responsibilities, many physicians accept shift work to relieve stress and have a more predictable work schedule. The day-to-day work is becoming more business-like; more income- and billing-driven; more documentation first and care second; more protocol-driven and less intellectual; and more data-driven with less quality patient interactions.

Technology changes are rapidly increasing throughout life. In addition to widely reported medical advances, the required documentation technology that now exists is becoming overwhelming. Besides reporting a patient's history, physical exam, and test results, the patient's medical chart must spell out the diagnostic plan, treatment expectations, and outcomes.

The electronic documentation of this required information is now in a state of constant flux, leading many physicians to change clinics in hopes of finding a more suitable work environment. While these doctors may appear less loyal to the patients and their partners, it is difficult to criticize their search for a system that is less corrosive to the physician-patient contract.

Sadly, this shift of focus from the patient to the process is leading to widespread physician burnout. For many doctors, after years of school and training programs, the "juice may no longer be worth the squeeze." This is especially true in neurology, which still has a limited therapeutic armamentarium (the medicines, equipment, and techniques available to a medical practitioner) to treat Alzheimer's Disease, ALS, and other inexorably progressive, incurable neurological conditions.

Besides being incurable, these neurological diseases often change the essence of a person, altering or destroying the very nature of what makes each human being unique. Watching the deterioration of one's patients day in and day out can be difficult, although not as devastating as it is to the family. Imagine the devastation for all concerned when a 90-year-old Minnesota man suffering from dementia shot and killed his caretaking son in the fall of 2015 (Pheifer & Walsh, 2015).

Summary

Numerous barriers currently prevent clinicians from practicing medicine as envisioned, as patients deserve, and as spelled out in the Hippocratic Oath. It is essential to return the physician's role to one of primarily interacting with patients. This will improve the accuracy of diagnosis and treatment choices. Reestablishing the primacy of the physician-patient interaction requires that clinicians spend less time justifying and documenting diagnostic and billing codes by delegating these bookkeeping tasks to others.

The future iterations of the EMR must live up to the initial promises to improve the efficiency of our system at a reasonable expense, allowing physicians to return to the bedside. Although trends toward large corporate group practice and subspecialization are unlikely to diminish, utilizing the input of practicing physicians will bring significant improvements.

Expanding the enrollment in medical schools and training programs while addressing the costs of education and physician financial incentives will aide doctor loyalty and job satisfaction, while decreasing physician mobility and the resulting fragmentation of care.

Epic changes are occurring at an increasingly rapid pace throughout society. Patient populations and physicians are not immune to these changes. Nonetheless, our healthcare system must remain true to its primary commitment of humane, patient-centered care for all at a reasonable expense.

On a positive note, the government is beginning to listen to physicians' concerns. A new five-year initiative called the "Comprehensive Primary Care Plus" (CPC+) model began in 2016 to "give doctors the freedom and flexibility to practice medicine the best way they know how, to return to what matters most to doctors and their patients" (Frieden, 2016).

Chapter 3
"Upside Down" Medical Care

All neurologists go through a similar process to become a Board Certified Neurologist. After medical school, they do a year of internship and three years of neurology residency before embarking on their life's mission and work. As is currently common throughout medicine, many physicians elect to spend another one to three years in fellowships to subspecialize. In neurology, these fellowships include:

- Vascular (stroke)
- Parkinson's Disease and movement disorders
- Alzheimer's Disease and dementia
- Pain
- Multiple Sclerosis
- Neuro-ophthalmology
- Autonomic disorders
- Neurophysiology
- Neuro-critical care
- Sleep
- Neuro-rehabilitation
- Concussion/brain and spinal cord trauma
- Neuro-behavioral disorders
- Neuro-oncology
- Epilepsy
- Neuro-palliative care

Despite the continual advancement of medical knowledge, training programs are now mandated to require fewer resident educational ("work") hours per week. To provide the equivalent educational experience in less hours per week, the programs would have to expand the years required to graduate. This has rarely occurred. Sensing their education and training is incomplete, graduating residents are electing to take fellowships to fill in the gaps in their training.

This subspecialization decision may also emanate from the physician being inspired by a specific disease, patient population, or desire to pursue a research project. Alternatively, the fellowship choice may be motivated by a wish to improve the physician's skill set and knowledge, allowing him to cope with the complexity and anxiety of keeping up with medicine's dramatic and rapid advances. To focus in depth on a smaller segment of the ever-expanding world of neuroscience may feel more comfortable.

The subspecialty training decisions are, in part, driven by physician marketability, interests of the senior staff members doing the training, and lifestyle considerations. Seldom is a Parkinson's Disease expert needed to analyze a medical emergency in the middle of the night. Reimbursement also favors subspecialty decisions.

While subspecialists have an important role to play in clinical medicine and in research, the numbers being produced are disproportionate to the need and further fragment patient care. As they learn more and more about less and less, subspecialists are highly trained to treat narrow segments of the population. Increasing the number of astute diagnosticians certainly is a credible goal. An unintended consequence is the subsequent decrease in the available pool of physicians with a wide range of knowledge. This limits the access to high-quality care for many patients. Unless many more physicians are trained, this is not a sustainable trend, as more clinicians spend longer training to treat smaller portions of the community.

To compensate, the medical schools and residencies must increase the number of students and trained physicians. Fortunately, the United States has seen a 25% increase in medical school enrollment between 2002-2003 and 2015-2016 to 21,434 students (Brooks, 2016). When combined with the increased enrollment in certified osteopathic medicine[10] colleges, this is indeed encouraging. Unfortunately, required graduate training programs for these medical students have not grown commensurately. Residencies and fellowships lack increased funding, including a long-standing cap on Medicare support (Brooks, 2016).

[10] A doctor of osteopathic medicine (D.O.) is a trained and licensed doctor who has completed similar residencies and is licensed identically to a medical doctor. He is also trained in "hands-on" manipulative treatments.

My daughter lived in Boston for ten years and had a difficult time finding a primary care doctor, despite Massachusetts having the largest number of physicians per capita in America (2015 State Physician Workforce Data Book). She eventually found a primary care nurse practitioner whose availability was limited to part-time office hours with after-hours coverage provided only by the emergency room.

The search for a physician will only become more problematic as the graying of America's baby boomers adds further demands on our delivery system, and our older general internists and family physicians retire. Approximately 50% of America's board-certified neurologists who typically practice general neurology are older than 55 years of age and are beginning to retire. They are being replaced with an ever-expanding array of subspecialists. A hospital administrator I know has observed a change in the work ethic in physicians today. He estimated that it would take 1.5 physicians to replace each retiring senior physician.

American healthcare gobbles up 18% of our GDP with mediocre results. The future requires wide access to high-quality "entry-level" care, not just top-end subspecialty services. One of the many reasons for our system providing inefficient and inconsistent care is that medicine is now, more than ever before, being practiced "upside down." This care model has been practiced at university medical centers for years, but is expanding into the community as subspecialization training has flourished.

Let me explain how this trend leads to added inefficiencies and added expenses in our already costly system. Everyone would agree that a well-organized system of medical care starts with a general medical practitioner who evaluates patients, treating appropriate cases and knowing when to refer to a specialist. For example, an internist identifies a possible neurological problem and refers the patient to a neurologist. The neurologist may, in turn, decide that the patient needs subspecialty expertise, such as a stroke neurologist, and engage the subspecialist as needed.

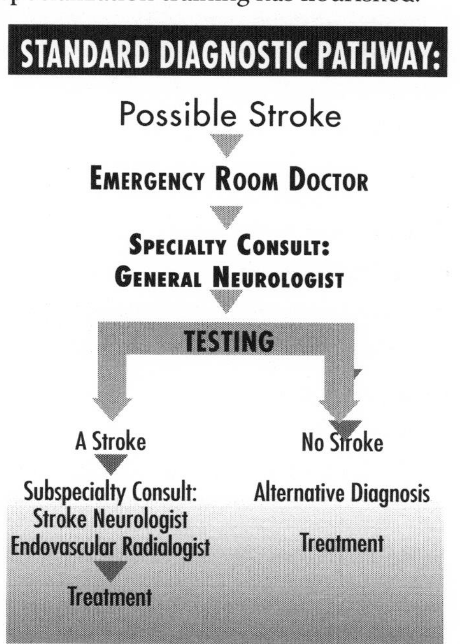

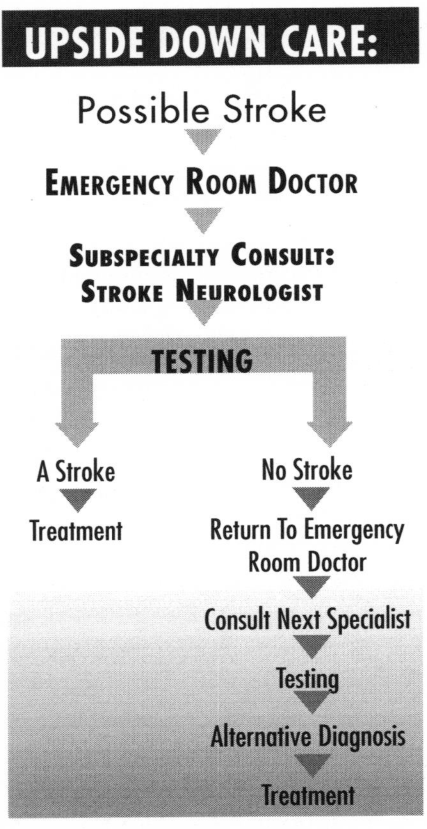

In an "upside down" system, the patient is triaged directly to the stroke neurologist. This is more likely to occur if general neurologists are in short supply and there is a plethora of subspecialists, such as stroke experts. Sometimes this works out well, saves a step, triggers an accurate diagnosis, and appropriate treatment is quickly and efficiently instituted. However, skipping steps may lead to mistakes and inefficiencies, as it does in many other arenas of life.

Short-circuiting the standard referral pathway runs the risk of starting in the wrong subspecialty, which then typically leads to unnecessary testing, while risking improper or delayed treatment. Even if it is fairly obvious to the subspecialist (in this case, the stroke neurologist) that the consult is inappropriate, she will typically feel the need to do testing to prove the patient's problem is not in her specialty area. If the testing for stroke is negative as expected, she may choose to refer the patient back "down" to the generalist, restarting the process after an expenditure of resources and time.

The subspecialists are many years removed from their original, more generalized specialty training (in this example, General Neurology). Knowing a great deal about a narrow set of illnesses, many fellowship-trained subspecialists choose not to venture outside of their subspecialty comfort zone, even though they were fully trained initially to do so. Our reimbursement system also encourages them to restrict the scope of their medical practice.

One of my fellow medical students became an internist with a subspecialty of oncology. He could, of course, discover cancer in a patient during an internal medicine consult. He joked that he could theoretically tell the patient, "I have bad news for you. You unfortunately have colon cancer. Additionally, the consult I just did now costs $10 more."

It turns out that subspecialists and generalists do not think through diagnostic puzzles similarly, as remarkable as that sounds. They literally have different routine approaches to diagnostic and therapeutic problems. The generalist considers a wide range of options when approaching a diagnostic quandary. A subspecialist, such as the stroke neurologist, typically approaches the patient predisposed to look for a diagnosis in her field.

The skill set of a subspecialist encompasses advanced, up-to-date knowledge about a narrow field of medicine, bringing it to the diagnostic and therapeutic process. She will view her job single-mindedly to identify a stroke, subsequently instituting timely, state-of-the-art treatment. When the subspecialist identifies the patient with one of the limited number of diagnoses in her subspecialty, she clearly adds value.

However, if the subspecialist deems the patient not to be suffering from a disease in her field, she likely will assume her job is done. Unfortunately, the patient is left with an unresolved medical problem. Often, after having extensive negative subspecialty testing, the patient may be discharged without a diagnosis with only a reassurance that nothing was found ("You did not have a stroke"). Alternatively, the diagnostic process can be started over again with a new referral. This scenario is what I have referred to as the "upside down" care model: Primary care to subspecialist . . . back to primary care . . . then to a different specialist/subspecialist.

In the most efficient medical care model, the key pivotal diagnostician is the generalist who is on "the front line." In contradistinction, because many of our healthcare networks currently employ a plethora of subspecialists and deemphasize the role of "front line" providers, inefficiencies and expenditures routinely increase.

When I began medical practice in neurology in the 1970s, many of the subspecialists continued to practice general internal medicine until their specialty practices grew. They approached patients as a subspecialist, yet remained concerned about the patient as a person with a problem, not only whether the diagnosis was in their field of expertise. I would regularly receive consults from them to consider if the medical quandary, such as abdominal pain, might have a neurological cause. As the entrenchment of subspecialists occurred in the last 25 years, these consults became more unusual. Rarely do gastroenterologists, for instance, having found no reason for a patient's abdominal pain, consider what the diagnosis might be outside their field of expertise. Having ruled out a problem in their field, they perceive their job as completed and "sign off" before the resolution of the patient's problem.

Summary

Few would disagree with the tenet that today's medical training programs should be based on the needs of the patient populations they serve. While ways exist for the government to influence the number of physicians trained in multiple medical fields, this guidance has not been sufficient to guarantee graduates in the fields that are most needed. The interests of the fellows and the senior staff have skewed the numbers of subspecialists, suggesting yet another example of our system focusing on the providers and not the patient.

Consequently, "upside down" care is becoming more prevalent throughout the country, no longer being restricted to the universities. This trend can hopefully be reversed with longer, more thorough general residencies, a revised reimbursement system that incentivizes a better care model, and a return to placing paramount importance on people in need.

Chapter 4
Healthy Lifestyle Choices: Stroke and Other Vascular Diseases

"If someone wishes for good health,
one must first ask oneself if he is ready to do away
with the reasons for his illness.
Only then is it possible to help him."

—Hippocrates

It is widely understood that a healthy lifestyle can decrease the occurrence and manifestations of disease, such as diabetes, hypertension, heart disease, and stroke. Consequently, for 40 years, my goal has been to urge patients to adopt healthy life choices. My efforts have encountered numerous barriers and excuses. One woman admitted that my suggestions on choosing a healthy lifestyle sounded too hard. She remarked, "How about something easier than a diet, like a temporary coma, which might function as a hard restart?"

Chapters 4 and 5 will focus on lifestyle change. **Chapter 4** considers recommendations for patients at risk for vascular disease, which is primarily stroke in neurological patients. **Chapter 5** considers recommendations for memory loss, dementia, headaches, epilepsy, Multiple Sclerosis, and Parkinson's Disease.

As a neurologist, who is also board certified as a Vascular Neurology Subspecialist,

I have dealt with a myriad of stroke patients. As with heart patients, stroke patients need to decrease their vascular risk factors to improve their health by incorporating lifestyle changes. Many of the modifiable vascular risk factors are interrelated and are more likely to be reduced with a wide array of healthy choices, not just, for instance, a diet alteration.

These changes should be routinely discussed in the doctor's office. The earlier in life a person embraces a healthy lifestyle, the easier it is to accomplish. These discussions become even more paramount when illness, such as a heart attack or stroke, has occurred. Education is important and motivation is key.

The institution of reasonable, simple, and realistic life changes are best and likely to be long-lasting. While short-term change is not without merit, long-term change is the goal. Physicians need to help patients establish a healthy lifestyle, not a diet that "I can go off of later." Having the support of family, friends, or a community can help facilitate change that will be long-lasting.

Getting Started

It is important for each person to start the process of change. A nice starting point for lifestyle counseling conversations is the American Heart Association (AHA) list of common modifiable vascular risk factors, called "Life's Simple Seven."

> ***"Prayer indeed is good, but while calling on the gods a man should himself lend a hand."***
> ***—Hippocrates***

1. No smoking.
2. Body Mass Index[11] less than 25 kg/m2.
3. Moderate exercise for at least 150 minutes per week or intense exercise for 75 minutes per week.
4. Incorporating four or five of the key components of an AHA healthy diet,[12] which encourages fruits, vegetables, fish, and whole grains, while discouraging animal fats, sweetened drinks, and sodium.

---

[11] Body Mass Index (BMI) is a measure of body fat based on height (in meters) and weight (in kilograms). For example, a man of 5'10" at 174 pounds has a BMI of 25 kg/m2 and a woman of 5'4" at 145 pounds has a BMI of 25 kg/m2. A BMI greater than or equal to 30 kg/m2 is considered obese.

[12] See number 8 under "Barriers to Healthy Eating" for the key components of an AHA healthy diet (page 68).

5. Total blood cholesterol level less than 200 mg/dL.
6. Blood pressure less than 120/80.
7. Fasting blood glucose less than 100 mg/dL (Paddock, 2010).

Patients can achieve significant benefits not just from physician-prescribed medications, but from personal choices like following Life's Simple Seven. Patients will also be advantaged by striving to decrease stress in their lives or altering their responses to stress. While we cannot avoid hereditary risk factors by choosing our relatives, we can make useful, healthy choices in how we live.

Although medications to lower blood pressure and cholesterol, control irregular heart rhythms, and "thin the blood"[13] can improve a person's chances to avoid a heart attack or a stroke, they are associated with a small but significant chance of complications, such as electrolyte imbalance, allergic reactions, muscle cramping, or bleeding ulcers. On the other hand, lifestyle changes are more difficult to maintain long term than taking a pill, but are effective and typically safe with few side effects.

As we all know, long-standing habits can be changed, but not easily. Indeed, we can choose to decrease stress in our lives. Alternatively, we can alter how we respond to the stresses in our lives. One of my patients happily bragged to me about getting off the fast track and adopting an effective mode of relaxation. She boasted that she was "the best at relaxing" of any of her friends, associates, and family members. Smiling, I wished her well, but I was not convinced that competing to be the best at relaxing was an example of truly stepping off the fast track.

Healthy Diet

As my father repeatedly pointed out, it is healthier "to eat to live, rather than live to eat." Unfortunately, few Americans abide by my dad's credo. Consequently, a significant portion of my patient counseling is focused on diet to minimize the risk of vascular disease, including stroke and heart attack.

> ***"Your foods shall be your 'remedies,' and your 'remedies' shall be your foods."***
> ***—Hippocrates***

[13] Medications that "thin the blood" typically slow the body's ability to form clots by changing the clotting factors (warfarin, for example) or decreasing the stickiness of the blood by interfering with platelet function (aspirin, for example).

It is becoming better known that a healthy diet includes fruits, vegetables, and nuts, while avoiding beef, sweetened drinks, saturated fats, and excessive salt. It is becoming increasingly accepted that not all fats and oils are created equal, although all are stocked with calories. Non-saturated fats are healthier than saturated fats (i.e. solid at room temperature) and trans fats. Oils with omega 3 and 6 are considered the most nutritious. Significant nutritional value exists in monounsaturated (i.e. liquid at room temperature, solid when chilled) and polyunsaturated oils, including olive, peanut, walnut, canola, grapeseed, sesame, and sunflower oils. It should be noted, however, that the more refined oils, like canola, have less antioxidants, decreasing their nutritional value.

> *"If we could give every individual the right amount of nourishment and exercise, not too little and not too much, we would have found the safest way to health."*
>
> *—Hippocrates*

The World Health Organization (WHO) announced in 2016 that a dramatic worldwide increase in diabetes had occurred during the last quarter-century (Keaten, 2016). The increase from 4.7% to 8.5% was driven by excessive weight gain, obesity, and aging. Dr. Margaret Chan, the WHO Director-General at that time, called for a worldwide increase in physical activity and healthy eating habits, highlighting the avoidance of foods and beverages high in sugar and fats.

My counseling of patients has focused primarily on obesity and the consumption of unhealthy foods that lead to strokes and heart disease. (I do not intend to dismiss anorexia as an important health issue, as indeed it can be fatal. However, as it is not a common vascular risk factor, anorexia is not typically addressed by neurologists.)

Barriers to Healthy Eating

Before listing common, reversible factors leading to obesity, it should be acknowledged that many causes of obesity, including inheritance, required medication usage, and illness, cannot be easily remedied by education and lifestyle alteration. Nonetheless, many people can be healthier by identifying and eliminating the following barriers to healthy eating. Clearly, as a newspaper article headline declared, "Weight loss isn't one size fits all" (Kolata, 2016).

Although it can be incredibly beneficial to eat healthy foods in appropriate portions, many barriers exist to adopting a new and healthier diet. Remarkably, it is estimated that Americans spend more money each year on potato chips than our universities spend on research. My patients have taught me that it is not easy to change. At an office visit, a patient, who failed her dieting goal and felt ashamed, looked at me and said, "Please do not look at me in that tone of voice, Dr. Schanfield." She and many of my other patients have led me to identify 16 common barriers to change.

1. Inaccurate self-perception: Most overweight individuals do not see themselves accurately. People seem to drop their weight category about one stage. For example, many overweight people think they are fine. Many obese people think they are overweight and may be insulted if referred to as obese. Many morbidly obese people will admit to being obese, but would be shocked to learn they are morbidly obese. As one patient explained, "I'm not obese. I just have a soft tissue surplus." Another obese man defended himself as "not fat, just thick."

2. Inertia: In life, inertia is a powerful phenomenon. We tend to feel safe and comfortable in long-established, familiar living habits and patterns. Even when these habits are clearly identified as unhealthy, the incentives to change often are insufficient to evoke action. One woman admitted it would be hard to change her diet: "That diet you recommended, doctor, sounds like 'a whatever I like to eat, don't eat it diet.'"

A morbidly obese man clearly not willing to invest the energy and time to change his diet remarked, "When a man has a large tool, he needs a big shed over it." Another man actually giggled and essentially changed the subject: "That's not my stomach. It's my bumper."

Some patients are without the will to consider change because of their age. An elderly woman who had suffered a small stroke was honest with me when I suggested that she should lose 20 pounds: "I'm not going to lose the 20 pounds you suggest. I'm going to take it with me . . . all the way.'"

3. Identity: Changes of long-established living patterns are especially difficult when they are firmly embedded in one's identity, especially if they have brought success and happiness. It may be unappealing to alter one's core behavior when it is the foundation of a person's self-worth. One patient, who identified himself as an excellent cook, remarked honestly, "I cannot possibly lose weight because I am a cook-aholic."

Other patients are high-energy, Type A individuals who are continually rewarded for living with crisis and stress. To step off the fast track and embrace a decrease in stress, improve sleeping and eating habits, and allow more time for exercise will likely lower blood pressure and minimize the possibility of premature heart disease and stroke. However, getting off the fast track may lead to depression and boredom with a decreased sense of purpose and self-worth. It may not be comfortable or easy to trade one's persona of "making the world go around" to one of contentedly "smelling the flowers."

4. Fast food: It has been well reported that fast food is readily available, cheap, great tasting, full of calories, and remarkably unhealthy. The ubiquitous availability of low-cost food with high-fat content is a significant barrier for many to embrace a healthy diet. Of all the food components, fats have the highest amount of calories per weight and may lead directly to developing atherosclerosis (hardening of the arteries), a primary contributor to heart disease and stroke.

Without clear understanding of how packed with calories, salt, and fat these foods are, a person may not understand their contribution to disease and obesity. As one sincere woman, who loved fatty foods, mistakenly remarked, "I don't eat too much. I'm an easy keeper. Whatever I eat seems to stay with me."

5. Sugar and corn syrup: Not only are fast foods cheap, readily accessible, and filled with fat and salt, many are loaded with corn syrup or sugar. Sweeteners sell and are popular. Corn syrup, being cheap, is now a widely used food additive for sweetness. It is now known that high fructose corn syrup, commonly used in soda pop, does not trigger the release of the satiety protein leptin. In other words, today's cola beverages and foods rich in high fructose corn syrup rarely satisfy a person's hunger.

It is now also well recognized that simple carbohydrates are metabolized very efficiently, triggering a rapid rise and then fall of blood sugar. This "yoyo" effect triggers a rebound hunger that also encourages overeating.

6. Social network: An individual's social network may impede one's ability to embrace new and healthier choices. In America, one can typically find a peer group to declare her alcohol and food consumption habits within the norm. The stigma of obesity has changed, with many social networks today actually promoting weight gain. I was fascinated when a patient understood the influence of his peer group, but spontaneously denied it with a smirk: "Our family does not believe in SCWG or

SCWL: socially contagious weight gain or socially contagious weight loss."

Peer groups should encourage healthy rather than unhealthy choices. Peer groups should encourage the ingestion of fruits, vegetables, and nuts. Examples are beginning to appear throughout the world of communities coming together to try to improve the health of their members by motivating healthy options and removing barriers to these options.

The city of Albert Lea, Minnesota, became a "blue zone" after the community leaders embraced Dan Buettner's concepts of healthy living and eating (2008). In 2009, Albert Lea began a community-wide approach to wellness by improving sidewalk and bike lanes. Restaurants were encouraged to offer a salad with a sandwich with an option of french fries, rather than the other way around. Within five years, Albert Lea had increased walking by 70% and decreased smoking by 4%. Participants in Albert Lea collectively lost almost four tons of weight (Walljasper, 2015).

7. Reasons we eat: Losing weight can be difficult if people eat despite not being hungry. Much of our eating is habitual, for comfort, or functions as a social activity. Years ago, I was surprised to learn that my eating habits were not necessarily the norm. While recovering from lumbar disc surgery, I overheard my wife talking to a friend on the phone. She said, "No, Paul has actually lost six to eight pounds since the surgery. He says that sitting around does not give him an appetite, so he's eating less the last few weeks." Shouting into the phone loud enough for me to hear across the room, her friend responded, "What does being hungry have to do with eating?"

It is typically enjoyable to eat good-tasting food, whether we are hungry or not. To maintain a healthy weight, a person must have a lifestyle that is not centered on eating. Many psychological issues and illnesses involve weight gain or weight loss. I have identified numerous patients who "stuff their emotions." When stressed, depressed, or anxious, they eat as a psychological defense mechanism, albeit an unhealthy one. One intermittently depressed woman explained to me, "Really, doctor, every now and then I do try to go on a diet."

8. Lack of information: Many people do not possess valid information concerning appropriate food choices. Learning what foods are unhealthy and packed with useless calories can lead some people to successfully change their habits. Some people are willing to be educated; some are not.

Even when motivated, nutritional science can be confusing to digest. What constitutes a healthy diet seems to be constantly evolving. Attempting to remain well informed, a person must remain vigilant to changes in nutritional theories and assumptions. As more information is presented clearly and simply, hopefully it will become easier for the American consumer to make wiser food and beverage choices.

In 2010, the American Heart Association published the key components of a healthy diet based on 2,000 calories a day:

1. 4.5 cups a day of fruits and vegetables
2. Two or more 3.5-ounce (100 grams) servings a week of fish (especially salmon or mackerel, which are high in omega-3 fatty acids)
3. Less than 450 kcal a week of sugar-sweetened beverages, with a 12-ounce can of cola equaling 139 kcal
4. Three or more one-ounce servings a day of whole grains, which are high in fiber and vitamins
5. Less than 1500 mg of sodium a day (Paddock, 2010)

9. Eating at the wrong time: Another barrier to a healthy lifestyle and better weight control is when we eat. It is now generally acknowledged that more physical activity after one's last meal each day correlates with fewer consumed calories stored by the body. Sumo wrestlers have learned this lesson. They strive to have prodigious physical strength and muscle mass, yet require enormous weight for leverage. They typically exercise all day and are fed all evening. They may not even stand after the last "feeding," rolling into bed from the table.

Patients should engage in some physical activity after eating and avoid eating right before sleep. Sadly, many dieters are careful all day, only to undo much of that good work with a late-night snack. These late-night snacks in front of the television allow most of the consumed calories to be converted directly to fat.

Other impediments to weight loss include eating very fast and following the famous credo of "eat dessert first." I presumed an overweight patient ate too fast when he admitted one should "always eat ice cream before it melts."

10. Seasons of loss: Another significant barrier to healthy eating for many of our elderly is living long enough to enter prolonged seasons of loss. They lose friends and family, leading to loneliness, depression, and hopelessness.

They also lose physical capabilities from ailments, such as arthritis, lung disease, and heart disease. This diminishes the amount of activity they can reasonably accomplish each day and decreases calories utilized. Despite gaining weight as she aged, a less mobile patient from a deteriorating spine was partially correct when she remarked, "I'm shrinking in height and I'm spreading out. So I'm not really overweight."

Many of my patients have retired after decades of productive, active life without carefully planning for the next stage of life. Becoming dramatically less active while maintaining the same dietary habits will predictably result in weight gain. Some retirees feel they "deserve" to eat what they want and be more inactive as they have "earned it."

11. Proliferation of medicines with weight gain side effects: In the last 30 years, it has become medically and socially acceptable to treat mood disturbances with psychotropic medicines rather than counseling, which can be long, cumbersome, and typically poorly reimbursed. These medications seem simple and safe. In reality, psychological health is more likely to be restored by a combination of "talk therapy," introspection, and medication.

Mood-altering medications are not as complication-free as once thought. Although not widely appreciated initially, it is now known that most of the psychologically active medications lead to weight gain. While clearly a factor in the obesity epidemic in America, this fact is rarely highlighted or discussed. Many people stay on these medications for years, long after the mood disturbance has cleared, not realizing that the medications may no longer be needed and may be a significant cause of their developing obesity.

Less prevalent, but also a problem, are other medications that have weight gain as a side effect. These include medications for diabetes, seizure disorders, beta blockers (to lower blood pressure and slow the heart rate), steroids (to suppress the immune system), and some pain pills.

12. Promise of diet pills: Another barrier is the hope for a "quick, easy fix." Many people prefer to find a medicine that will allow them to eat what they want and still lose weight. After curing cancer or Alzheimer's Disease, surely some people would consider an effective, side effect-free weight loss drug as the Holy Grail of medicine. Whereas no evidence exists that diet pills prolong or improve life, they are very popular, yet can be dangerous. The pills have a small but definite risk of cardiac disease, cancer, addiction potential, and cognitive issues.

Between 2013-2015, in just three years, the FDA approved five new weight-loss medications after intense lobbying by the pharmaceutical corporations, congress, medical societies, and their constituents. Despite being so popular, these drugs only promise losses of 5% to 10% of body weight. Even if the promised weight loss is realized, this amount of weight loss has little proven benefit, unless it is viewed as the beginning of a long-term lifestyle change.

13. Yoyo diets: As mentioned above, the key to long-term health is to adopt a healthy lifestyle, centered on maintaining a vigorous activity level and a reasonable diet. Instead, many patients opt for dramatic diet programs that are neither sustainable nor healthy. Although patients on these diets experience impressive weight loss in the short term, they unfortunately regain the lost pounds in the future. Their weights yoyo from year-to-year.

Jane Brody, a health columnist for *The New York Times*, put it beautifully when she spoke to a group of doctors in the Twin Cities: "Most Americans go on a diet, so that they can go off it later. . . . It is now time in America to stop the rhythm method of girth control."

14. Stress, depression, and/or poor sleep: It is becoming more widely appreciated that poor sleep leads to weight gain. In addition, it is almost too obvious to mention that psychological illnesses and stress interfere with normal, healthy patterns of eating, activity, and sleep, often leading to unhealthy weight changes. If a previously healthy person begins to develop weight issues without apparent cause, issues of stress, sleep, or possible psychological illness should be carefully explored.

15. Lack of physical activity: Inherent in a number of these barriers is the fact that many Americans today do not maintain adequate physical activity, especially as they age. A slowing of metabolism seems to occur with age. Therefore, we should decrease the caloric intake or increase the amount of regular physical exercise as we age, preferably both.

Most Americans seem to do the opposite. Thinking out loud, one man stated, "I regularly exercise . . . well, sort of in spurts . . . occasionally . . . actually, not very often." To some extent, this can be unavoidable with the aging of the body, developing physical limitations (mentioned above), and the increasing demands and responsibilities of adulthood. It is certainly possible, however, for many aging people to make the appropriate lifestyle changes once they become aware of the consequences from a lack of regular physical activity.

16. Excuses: Many of my overweight patients, with seemingly good nature, make excuses that actually undermine their ability to change:

- "It turns out I have an elbow flexion-mouth reflex. With elbow flexion, my mouth drops open and swallowing kicks right in."
- "I was put on a cardiac diet, but my heart was not into it."
- "Thinovation. Ha, ha, ha . . . I don't believe in that."
- "I'm just a salt-aholic. Nothing serious."
- "I'm a bread-aholic, but I can otherwise easily change my diet."
- "My obesity is not inherited. It is due to my free-range eating habits."
- "Brains come and go, but fat cells live forever."
- "I am a high-calorie eater."
- "I am a volume eater; I could eat right through bariatric surgery."

Keys to healthy eating

Even though these barriers are indeed powerful in preventing lifestyle change, I have used a few simple tenets to help my patients break through these habits and excuses and change their diets effectively.

> *"It is safer to proceed a little at a time, especially when changing from one regimen to another."*
> *—Hippocrates*

To reduce one's weight over the long term, doctor and patient need to discuss a few key factors:

Motivation: Most important, patients need to have a sincere motivation and commitment to change their lifestyle.

Plan: A plan must be established that is easy to follow, incorporates long-term dietary changes, and includes regular outcome assessments. In addition, the plan should be individualized for each person, as people may respond differently to the same diet plan.

Lifestyle, not just diet: Because weight loss is not determined only by eating habits, a successful diet needs to be coupled with addressing one's physical activity and habits. In other words, the lifestyle as a whole needs to be fundamentally and permanently addressed.

Supportive social network: People need to be in a social network that will encourage these choices over the long term.

A success story is an 83-year-old woman patient of mine who lost 22 pounds in eleven months. The only change that led to this rather significant weight loss was that her daughter, with whom she lived, eliminated her late night snack of two or three cookies from her diet. When she was seen by me in the office, the lovely and slimmer woman did not even remember that her daughter had taken her cookies away. A long-term habit was altered by a favorable social network and turned out to be easily sustainable.

Activity and Exercise

> *"Sport is the preserver of health."*
> *—Hippocrates*

While a sedentary existence leads to obesity, it is also a vascular risk factor in and of itself. The average American does so little physical movement during the day that he loses 1% of his muscle mass each year after 30 years of age. Gretchen Reynolds, Phys Ed columnist for *The New York Times*, reported that "regular walking, cycling, swimming, dancing, and even gardening" may substantially reduce the risk of vascular disease and Alzheimer's Disease (Reynolds, 2016).

Increasing the physical activity in modern life turns out to be more difficult to alter than I had naively thought at the start of my career. My patients will joke with me about their lack of exercise: "No, I did not sign up for Tai Chi like you recommended. I thought it was a fancy tea."

Many people just do not have the motivation to alter their activity level. "Whenever I get the urge to exercise," expressed one of my patients, "I lie down and rest till it passes." Remarkably, even during an office visit, I get pushback for suggesting activity. For example, after asking a patient to get up and walk to the examining room door and back, she responded, "All in one day, doctor?"

When trying to increase a person's routine, the added daily physical activity should be non-threatening and doable. Effective activity does not have to be strenuous, but the commitment must have long-term traction. Increasing the physical requirements of routine activities can burn calories while improving muscle tone and bulk as we age. We can choose not to park in the closest parking spot. We can choose to take the stairs instead of the elevator.

I learned early in my career to encourage simple increases in physical activity. For instance, many people nowadays use an electric toothbrush that runs for two minutes. I tell my patients that, instead of standing in front of the mirror in the bathroom, they can use those two minutes (two to three times each day) to do some type of simple exercise. I use the two-minute periods to stretch my muscles and balance on one foot, then the other. I encourage my elderly patients to, each time they stand or sit, do so three times. This increase in activity is simple, easy, sustainable, and effective.

Scheduling regular exercise is another tenet of long-term change. Many well-meaning people plan to exercise at the end of the day after all other tasks have been completed. By that time, I commonly hear that "I was just too tired to work out" or "It's hard to get to sleep after exercising late at night." Setting a specific time dedicated to exercise is more likely to succeed.

Remarkably, most people become energized after physical exercise, which helps perpetuate exercise over the long term. Therefore, it is important to start. Once beginning a realistic routine, real change has the best chance of being achieved.

In Manchester, England, a new initiative has taken hold. The city developed an "older people's play area," featuring six pieces of equipment with the slogan, "Never too old to play." The area is designed to provide gentle exercise (Over-70s Only! Manchester Opens Playground for Oldies, 2008). As the Manchester community obviously believes, having a safe, easily accessible, and appealing place to exercise is an advantage. It is exciting to imagine that an initiative like Manchester's might succeed and be replicated around the world.

Besides having an attractive place, a reasonable plan, and a regular schedule, increased commitment to successful change is aided by exercising with other people. This increases one's ongoing commitment through socialization and peer pressure. Few people want to disappoint friends or family members.

If one cannot exercise with another person, many success stories begin with buying a dog, who happily encourages walks twice each day. Of course, no approach is foolproof. An elderly patient acquired a dog he faithfully walked 30 to 60 minutes each day. "The dog looks great," he said, "although I have not lost any weight." It turned out the man treated himself to additional "deserved" snacks because of his dog walking while the dog's diet remained the same.

Another approach is to join a health club, because paying for membership is often a motivating factor to follow through with the exercise program. This, too, can generate an excuse. One patient explained to me that the membership to the health club was too expensive: "It costs $100 every time I walk into the club." When I looked at her skeptically, she admitted, "The club had a $200 initiation fee and cost $33 a month thereafter. I went three times in three months, doc."

Although no exercise or physical activity is free from risk of injury, the scientific data suggests it is worth the risk as "movement is medicine." While "physical inactivity is a primary cause of many of the chronic ailments which afflict an aging population," physical activity is usually beneficial. "Physical activity sets off a cascade of signals which, if repeated, improve the function of our body and brain, diminishing the risk of cardiovascular disease and metabolic disorders, reducing anxiety, and enhancing concentration and attention" (Hewitt, 2017).

Some people seem to be programmed to expend more energy during life than others and maintain a healthy weight regardless of their diet. My personal trainer, Jocey, introduced me to the concept of NEAT, which stands for non-exercise activity thermogenesis. Dr. J. A. Levine from the Mayo Clinic defines NEAT as a measurement of "the energy expended for everything we do that is not sleeping, eating, or sports-like exercise. It ranges from the energy expended walking to work, typing, performing yard work, undertaking agricultural tasks, and fidgeting" (Levine, 2002, pp. 679-702).

In other words, people who fidget often are skinnier than those who are more typically in repose. Presumably, our individual brains uniquely control our metabolism, trying to keep our weight stable if we overeat or significantly restrict our intake. If we understood how this regulation worked, we might more readily be able to counsel patients on how to achieve and sustain a healthier body size.

Smoking

It is well known that smoking can be a modifiable risk factor for stroke, heart disease, lung disease, and cancer. The multiple avenues that are now available to aid in quitting are also well known. Despite Americans smoking less, many patients remain hopelessly addicted. A patient, who found it too hard to quit, explained, "I know that smoking may take ten years off my life, but it will invariably be the last ten. They are often not that good anyway, doc."

Some patients have indeed "cut back" in the amount they smoke, which is not without benefit. It is not an empty excuse to declare, "I'm only a recreational smoker." When I began practicing neurology in the mid-1970s, doctors' lounges were commonly filled with smokers. I was rather skeptical when the hospitals began moving to become smoke-free, yet it has happened. Even more remarkable has been the passing of laws requiring restaurants, bars, and public buildings to be smoke-free in Minnesota and 33 other states.

A great deal of social pressure continues to exist for minimizing smoking. Except for the young and the restless, smoking rates are at an all-time low and are unlikely to accelerate again.

Alcohol

> ***"Who could have foretold, from the structure of the brain, that wine could derange its functions?"***
> ***—Hippocrates***

Alcohol use in moderation, which can be healthy and enjoyable, is common across the globe. As a matter of fact, red wine is now known to have some positive health values. Yet, established long-term habits can be difficult to modify. I suggested that an elderly widower sometimes switch his daily beer to a glass of red wine. Scowling, he responded, "I'd prefer to drink panther piss than red wine."

However, drinking alcohol can get out of hand and lead to the destruction of a person's life and family. Like smoking, the ravages of excessive alcohol are now commonly understood. As one man put it, "I'm allergic to alcohol; if I drink too much, I break out in handcuffs."

It is less well known that alcohol is rich in calories. Only fat has more calories by weight than alcohol. For some patients, alcohol consumption may be a hidden source of calories. Of course, I have heard my share of alcohol-related excuses and jokes, such as, "So, doctor, how big is this only one alcoholic beverage I'm allowed each day?"

Serious problems erupt when a person becomes dependent upon an ever-increasing amount of alcohol. Like being overweight or inactive, my patients tend to joke about their use of alcohol. One patient wrote in his history form: "Smoking: No; Alcohol: As needed." Another patient filled out his history form by writing, "Alcohol: As much as I want."

Fortunately, many patients respond appropriately to their families' concerns and limit their alcohol consumption. A quick-witted man remarked that he takes his pills in his shot glass, "because that is the only thing that my wife will allow me to put in it."

Summary

No one disagrees that lifestyle choices can have a significant influence on life and illness. However, to succeed in causing effective and substantial lifestyle change, a great deal of work needs to be done by the physician and the patient. As opposed to taking a pill, the patient's "work" is often not simple or easy, requiring personal changes be maintained over the long term. This chapter reviewed my approach to counseling and educating patients to minimize the risk of vascular disease, including heart attack and stroke.

> ***"The patient must combat the disease along with the physician."***
> ***—Hippocrates***

When asked how she remains alive and vigorous at 92 years of age, a patient of mine responded, "A person must always eat right and move their butt. You sit, you die."

Chapter 5

Healthy Lifestyle Choices: Other Neurological Conditions

Treating stroke and other vascular diseases by altering a person's lifestyle, as examined in the previous chapter, emphasized the significance of individual responsibility. Information is accumulating that a person's life choices can influence the course of many other medical conditions, including memory loss, dementia, headache, epilepsy, Multiple Sclerosis, and Parkinson's Disease. This chapter explores these conditions and how a patient's lifestyle can influence them.

Memory Loss

As the population ages, the onset of dementia is becoming a major public health concern. It is estimated that 10,000 people will turn 65 years of age each year for many years to come (Bernard, 2012). Not surprisingly, increasing numbers of aging patients come to physician offices concerned about memory loss.

"The Worried Well": It is clearly a neurologist's job to address whether these memory loss concerns are a manifestation of dementia, such as Alzheimer's Disease, or are benign concerns of "the worried well." The worried well include the vast majority of patients who come to the office on their own, complaining of memory loss. They are not suffering from illness, merely noticing the consequences of normal aging. Their mere recognition of these changes typically indicates they are not ill. However, dementia patients lose this type of insight as the illness robs them of executive functioning prior to developing memory loss and word finding.

A person who can learn does not have dementia, even if he manifests word-finding issues, slowed reaction and retrieval times, complex attention issues, and visuospatial declines. While relatively minor cognitive and memory issues occur with age, healthy seniors have the ability to place new memories in context (the big picture) which far outweighs the losses, leading to the possibility of a continued accumulation of wisdom. Approximately 80% of 80-year-olds function normally.

Reassurance is not always well-received, of course. A charming woman honestly admitted, "You told me to stop worrying and I appreciate that, but you might as well tell me to stop breathing, doc."

Dementia: Dementia is a progressive decline in cognitive abilities caused by disease that interferes with a person's ability to function normally. Those who are truly demented lack appropriate insight and are typically brought to the clinic by their family. An example of dementia is an accountant whose staff or family realizes that she is spending more time getting less done. Although she can perform the appropriate calculations, she has developed difficulty judging when the tax forms are correct and finished.

Each patient deserves a thorough investigation for a cure when diagnosed as having dementia. A small percentage of patients have a reversible cause of the dementia. Examples include:

- Hypothyroidism.
- A benign space occupying mass in the skull (like a chronic subdural hematoma, benign brain tumor, or large cyst).
- Vitamin deficiency (like B1 or B12 deficiencies).
- A sleep disturbance that deprives the brain of oxygen (like sleep apnea).
- A subacute/chronic central nervous system infection.

The most common disease that causes dementia is Alzheimer's Disease, which has no known cure. Vascular disease of the brain is the second most common entity leading to forgetfulness. It is now apparent that vascular disease and Alzheimer's Disease commonly coexist, so lifestyle changes should be adjusted for both.

In 2010, five million Americans suffered from dementia. That number is predicted to grow dramatically as the graying of America continues, possibly tripling by 2050. However, the Framingham Heart study[14] documents the hopeful finding that the average age of the onset of dementia has increased from 80 years of age to 85 years of age since the 1970s (Belluck, 2016).

The development of dementia can be documented by memory testing. However, memory loss is not ordinarily the first intellectual domain to suffer in dementia. More complicated, higher cortical functions of cognition become disrupted before identifiable memory loss occurs.[15] Judgment, abstract reasoning, insight, and other executive-type intellectual processes are likely to decline earlier than memory and may inhibit a person's insight into the illness.

While many demented patients tend to have some hint that they are having cognitive issues, impaired insight and judgment typically prevents meaningful comprehension of the condition. Therefore, neurologists depend heavily on family, friends, and coworkers for more accurate historical observations, insights, and opinions. If the diagnosis is in question, of course, formal testing is performed, including neuropsychometric testing that typically lasts 2-4 hours.

Treatment and prevention of dementia: As mentioned above, no cures exist for most dementia patients, but many useful treatment approaches can be prescribed, including a healthier lifestyle, medications, education, and diet. For females, living with another person, having volunteer activities, being married, and experiencing frequent social visits with family, friends, and neighbors "often predicted memory resilience" (Greb, 2016, p. 14). Oddly, for men, the only predictor of memory resilience in one study was less depressive symptoms (Greb, 2016, p. 14).

Medications: Although no cures for Alzheimer's Disease currently exist, Dr. Jin-Tai Yu and colleagues at the University of California San Francisco found vitamin supplements may be helpful with some meta-analysis information, suggesting that folate, Vitamin E, and Vitamin C may be protective (Peckel, 2016). Research is

---

[14] The Framingham Heart Study is a large collection of health information that began in 1948 with participants from Framingham, Massachusetts. Researchers continue to follow all participants and periodically publish longitudinal epidemiological results.

[15] The cerebral cortex is a layer of gray matter (neurons) that covers the cerebral hemispheres and is responsible for higher functions of the brain, including learning, language, memory, integration of voluntary muscle activity, and the recognition of sensory inputs (smell, touch, hearing, tasting and vision).

continuing concerning the efficacy of Vitamin D. I should note that "no dietary supplement, not ginseng, Ginkgo biloba, omega-3, or coconut oil, has been scientifically proven to boost brain function or thwart cerebral decline" (Avitzur, 2016, p. 6).

In addition, some evidence is accumulating from large meta-analysis studies that suggests exposure to estrogen, statin medications that lower cholesterol, antihypertensive medications, and nonsteroidal anti-inflammatory therapies may help protect against developing Alzheimer's Disease (Peckel, 2016).

The FDA has approved medications for Alzheimer's Disease. These prescriptions partially improve symptoms for a short time for some patients, while failing to address the underlying disease condition. Because of the limited effectiveness of these medications, much research is being done to hopefully develop better medications.

An example from one of my patients illustrates the limited scope of effectiveness of the current medications. I started this patient on one of the approved medications. Upon returning to the clinic, his wife announced that he was somewhat improved, although he seemed unchanged to me. I asked her for an example of his improvement. She was able to give me two different observations:

- First, he was more confident and would answer the phone, taking messages that he had avoided in the past several months.
- Secondly, his wife felt he could better help with kitchen chores. She explained that they were married later in life and when "you marry late in life, the men tend to come better trained." She went on to explain that when they dined at home together, they did the dishes together; one person washing, while the other dried. "Sadly, his decline had restricted him to only dishwashing. Since taking the new Alzheimer's medication, he could once again dry the dishes." Mystified, I inquired as to what this had to do with his memory problems. Smiling, his wife explained that the dryer also put the dishes away and he had forgotten where they went. "This last month," she remarked, "he can again remember and I'm so pleased." Because the medication provides a symptomatic boost at best, the inexorable progression of the condition eliminated this improvement after about six months.

Modifiable Dementia risk factors: A 2016 Neurology Review article listed seven risk factors that, if modified, could possibly prevent or delay the onset of dementia: physical inactivity, depression, midlife hypertension, midlife obesity, smoking, low educational attainment, and diabetes (Day). Because the evaluation and treatment of depression, hypertension, smoking, and diabetes are relatively straightforward, I will explore physical inactivity, education, and diet as they relate to the development of dementia.

1. Physical inactivity: A physician's first step in the treatment of dementia is to emphasize healthy choices that include a heart-healthy diet, as much physical activity as possible, an expanded social network, and efforts to enhance mental capacities to the fullest. With the recent insight that vascular changes often coexist with Alzheimer's Disease, focusing on good vascular health can be helpful. Lowered blood pressure, a good night's sleep, and physical exercise, even if started in middle age, may protect against cognitive decline (Avitzur, 2016).

Maria Carrillo, chief science officer for the Alzheimer's Association,[16] expresses "hope for Alzheimer's if a push for healthier lifestyles accompanies efforts to find treatments" (Belluck, 2016). Dallas Anderson, a dementia program director at the National Institute of Aging, also sets a positive tone by emphasizing that each of us can "take steps to postpone" the clinical manifestations of Alzheimer's Disease (Avitzur, 2016, p. 6).

Dr. Michael Rosenbloom, the clinical director of the HealthPartners Center for Memory and Aging in St. Paul, extols the virtues of healthy lifestyle choices: "We know those who are more physically active, those who are socially active—these are also protective factors against developing dementia later in life" (Shah, 2015).

2. Education: Recent information suggests that education may slow the development of dementia symptoms. Pam Belluck reviewed a 2016 New England Journal of Medicine article "which provides the strongest evidence yet that better education and cardiovascular health are contributing to a decline in new dementia cases over time, or at least helping more people stave off dementia for longer" (Belluck, 2016). Therefore, continuing to embrace education as we age should be strongly encouraged.

Continued intellectual curiosity and involvement in learning tends to decline with age, but I urge my patients to resist this decline. Continued learning may, Belluck suggests, "generate neural connections, allowing brains to compensate longer when memory and thinking falter" (2016). I encourage patients to take up new hobbies and other intellectual pursuits.

---

[16] Alzheimer's Association is an advocacy group, which also funds research.

I encourage patients to continue enriching their social activities and connections, because it follows logically that physical, mental, and social withdrawal leads to more rapid decline of brain functioning. I should note that I attempt to "practice what I preach." I organize monthly bridge games, participate in a couple's book club, and have developed a monthly "Guys' Movie Night Out."

Just as with one's body, "use it or lose it" pertains to the mind. "It is very reasonable to recommend that our patients remain cognitively and socially engaged, whatever that means for the individual patient" (Day, 2016, p. 21). A recent study "concluded that older adults who had a mentally stimulating lifestyle and limited their consumption of unhealthy foods appeared to be at the least risk of dementia, compared with other participants" (Robinson, 2016b, p. 38)

However, "there is no clear demonstration of benefit of cognitive training, nor is there evidence to suggest that one cognitive training strategy is better than another" (Day, 2016, p. 21). In 2016, Lumos Labs, the marketer of Luminosity, a computer- and app-based brain training program, agreed to pay two million dollars to redress misleading advertising claims that the "program would sharpen performance in everyday life and protect against cognitive decline" (Federal Trade Commission, 2016).

3. Diet: A recent study listed "adherence to a Western dietary pattern (e.g., consumption of red and processed meats, potatoes, white bread, and prepackaged foods and sweets) . . . as a poor diet" (Robinson, 2016b, p. 38). Evidence is accumulating that a healthy diet, like the Mediterranean Diet, in addition to decreasing vascular disease of all types, may directly "protect aging brains from dementia" (Shah, 2015). This is a diet rich in olive oil, fish, nuts, fruits, and fresh vegetables.

Susan Fitzgerald reviewed a Rush University study that found that the brain is protected when a person possessing the APOE e4 gene, a gene known to increase the risk of Alzheimer's Disease, eats at least one seafood meal a week (Fitzgerald, 2016). Eating fish carries the potential harm of increasing the amount of mercury in the body, which can act as a poison. However, the Rush University researchers found no increase in brain pathology related to the mercury accumulation (Morris et al., 2016).

Even dessert might be potentially healthy. Evidence now exists that cocoa flavonoid in dark chocolate may penetrate and accumulate in the brain regions associated with learning and memory. This key component in dark chocolate may also promote nerve cell growth and enhanced blood flow to the brain (Dark Chocolate

Found to Offer Brain Health Benefits, 2015).

Headaches

As with stroke, vascular disease, and memory loss, headache patients can mitigate their symptoms with lifestyle changes, especially when suffering from tension and migraine headaches.

Tension headaches: Most people have headaches from time to time, leading to headache being the most common problem seen in medical clinics. Successful headache treatments begin with the correct diagnosis, with tension headaches leading the list of potential diagnoses. Interestingly, once the diagnosis of muscle tension headache is confirmed, sufficient patient anxiety may be relieved to improve the pain syndrome, without the need for other treatment modalities. However, I am sure it does not come as a surprise to suggest that tension headache patients can benefit from lifestyle changes.

Not infrequently, people lack insight concerning how stress can cause their specific physical complaints, like headaches. I recall a striking example of a 28-year-old woman with one month of headaches. She was physically normal, leading me to diagnose tension headaches that often emanate from stress. She disturbingly denied any such stress. My family practice medical resident and I talked about the case at length. We were both unenthusiastic about invasive testing to rule out a serious medical condition, but uneasy diagnosing a tension headache without any contributory history of stress or tension.

We elected to have the medical resident retake the patient's history. With just the female medical resident in the room, the patient revealed that she moved out of her home a month before, when her husband and his girlfriend moved in. Amazingly, this lovely, young woman had not related her headaches to her marital crisis. She knew about the girlfriend and said, "I'm fine with it. I'm over it," as she burst into tears.

Stress can lead to muscle tension in the scalp and the neck. Stress can lead to poor sleeping and eating. Stress can lead to anxiety and depression. All of these factors must be addressed and treated, if possible, to relieve the headache syndrome. Ideally, the stress should be eliminated, for example, by leaving an abusive boss and finding a new job.

If the stress can't be easily eliminated, the patient's response to the stress should then be analyzed and hopefully improved. This may involve counseling, a new exercise program, a healthy diet, an evaluation of sleep habits, the institution of new coping mechanisms, or applying a good dose of common sense.

One effective way to cope with muscle tension is to master biofeedback relaxation exercises. During biofeedback training, the patient learns to identify muscle tension, often in the scalp, face, and neck muscles. In my experience, learning biofeedback is often preferable to treating pain with habit-forming medications and passive physical therapy modalities, like massage and ultrasound.

Sometimes physical therapy and medications can be effective if utilized only temporarily, much like Band-Aids. Breaking the headache cycle can reduce the patient's anxiety by proving the pain syndrome is indeed benign.

The danger of these passive, Band-Aid treatments is that they merely cover up the underlying problem of stress, which continues to fester. This approach is typically ineffective and may lead to a long-term dependence on ever-increasing doses of medications.

This medication dependency is well known with narcotics, but is less recognized when caused by over-the-counter pain medications (for example, Tylenol, Aspirin, and Advil). Physicians refer to this phenomenon as the "over-the-counter, overuse medication headache syndrome." In this syndrome, clearly "less is more."

> ***"To do nothing is sometimes a good remedy."***
> ***—Hippocrates***

Migraine headaches: Migraine headache is the second most common headache syndrome. Excellent medications exist to both alleviate an acute migraine attack and prevent attacks.

The first step in treating migraines is to determine if the patient is inadvertently on a medication that may exacerbate the migraines. The classic example is female hormones, such as birth control pills, which are known to trigger migraine headaches in susceptible individuals. Fortunately, a lower dose of estrogen in "the pill" may still be effective birth control, yet trigger less headaches.

Once a physician diagnosis of migraine is identified, the second step in treating migraines is patient education, including the identification of individual headache triggers. The third step is to prescribe appropriate medications, while explaining that medicines to abort migraine attacks are also susceptible to overuse and rebound.

Migraines can be so painful as to encourage the overuse of migraine medications. The overuse of these medications is often triggered by the fear of suffering a bad migraine, leading patients to take them early and often. This may lead to withdrawal and rebound medication-induced headaches, which are often indistinguishable from the migraines themselves, complicating the treatment dramatically.

Besides appropriate pharmacological treatment, education, and avoidance of overmedication, migraine headache sufferers can do several things to prevent migraines that are lifestyle-based. Diet manipulation is important as a number of foods clearly trigger migraine attacks, especially if they have added chemicals, such as nitrites, nitrates, and MSG. In many patients, too much salt in their diet may increase the likelihood of migraine headaches. Skipping meals can also trigger headaches, as can some alcoholic beverages, especially red wine.

As with tension headaches, stress, poor sleep, and inadequate physical exercise can increase the frequency of migraine headaches. In one study, 80% of the patients reported stress as the most common trigger of their migraines (Robinson, 2016a). A rather interesting phenomenon unique to migraine sufferers is the "let-down" attack. In this scenario, the migraine occurs after the stress has passed. For example, a person completes two weeks of work in one week so that she can go on vacation. The migraine onset can be delayed, striking the patient when on vacation.

A final, important note about migraine headache patients: For migraineurs, it is my experience that headache is their "Achilles heel," their "weak spot" and physical sign of stress. As the years pass, the majority of migraine sufferers develop tension headaches. To complicate their situation further, it is common for a tension headache to trigger a migraine attack. In these cases, the neurologist's task includes teaching the patient to differentiate accurately between a tension headache and a migraine attack, and then treat each one appropriately.

> ***"The natural force within each of us is the greatest healer of all."***
> ***—Hippocrates***

Without the ability to clearly differentiate a tension headache from a migraine, an uneducated patient will likely overuse medications, often trying both migraine pills and tension headache pills in frustration. This is yet another path to the development of disabling rebound headaches, leaving these unfortunate patients to suffer three unique headache syndromes simultaneously, each with a different optimum treatment regimen. How miserable and confusing for a person to have rebound headaches superimposed upon migraines and tension headaches. In my experience, these patients are often surprised to learn that the key to feeling better is less medication. Once again, "less is more."

Multiple Sclerosis and Parkinson's Disease

While Multiple Sclerosis and Parkinson's Disease are two very different illnesses, they are both good examples of chronic, progressive neurological conditions not caused by unhealthy lifestyle choices. Nonetheless, lifestyle choices can still be important to patients suffering from these conditions.

One day, my schedule was filled with MS and Parkinson's patients complaining of progressive weakness, despite being medically stable. The answer to this conundrum became clear to me when I delved deeper into their daily routines. Each of the patients were allowing their chronic neurological diseases to dictate the pace of their life. They were more sedentary than necessitated by their disability. They had not given up, but they had unwittingly prematurely surrendered their lives to the illness. After being sedentary for months to years, they indeed were weaker, in large part due to disuse, not from disease.

Neurologists are taught to focus on medications, disease symptoms, and abnormal signs found on the physical exam. Yet, that day I realized it is important to also focus on the details of patients' day-to-day existence, not just the manifestations of their illness. Since having this epiphany, I have routinely counseled each patient to be as physically and mentally active as is reasonably safe. I counsel patients to take charge of their lives and their diseases. Each patient hopefully leaves our office with a realistic understanding of the amount of regular exercise and activity that is appropriate. This is the best way I have found to delay premature weakness and disability.

I tell my patients that if they cannot run, then they should walk. If they cannot walk, they should ride a bike. If they cannot bike safely outside, they should use a stationary bike, elliptical trainer, rowing machine or some other piece of stationary equipment indoors. If they cannot navigate such exercise equipment, they should stand as much as possible. If they cannot stand, they should exercise their legs and their arms while sitting.

> ***"Walking is a man's best medicine."***
> ***—Hippocrates***

Sometimes, of course, patients with debilitating physical illnesses tend to overdo and embark on unsafe activities. Because falls can be devastating setbacks, physical activity must be done safely. However, at times, counseling patients with balance issues to use walking aids has been complicated by their embarrassment to do so.

One man was particularly obstinate in his refusal to accept a cane. Sporting a big grin, he walked in my office one day using a golf putter like a walking stick, carrying it upside down. He looked at me and said, "I have begun carrying this putter only partially for balance, as I am now the only person around who can respond if an emergency putt is required."

The topic of individuals continuing in unsafe activities with chronic illness was the theme of a *Neurology* editorial by Dr. Zachary Simmons. Commenting on the Stephen Hawking film, *The Theory of Everything,* Simmons claimed:

> I am not at all certain that age brings wisdom, but it certainly brings perspective and experience. In the end, all of us, even when limited by a devastating illness, must engage in those activities that bring value to our lives, or life is not worth living. I can provide advice, but ultimately patients must seek a compromise between a meaningful and potentially dangerous life, and one that is safer but less meaningful (2015, p. 2079).

Epilepsy

We now have a much clearer understanding of what causes seizures than in the time of Hippocrates. No longer do we consider epilepsy divine intervention or witchcraft. Being a chronic, paroxysmal disease characterized by seizures triggered by abnormal electrical brain discharges, it can often be controlled, although rarely cured. Epilepsy is, therefore, an excellent example of a chronic medical condition typically requiring long-term medication.

To be sure, it is important for epileptics to have a healthy lifestyle, such as avoiding sleep deprivation, stress, and excessive alcohol intake, especially binge drinking. Furthermore, it is of paramount importance for patients with epilepsy to faithfully take their medications precisely as prescribed, which is seldom easy.

> *"Men think epilepsy divine, merely because they do not understand it. We will one day understand what causes it, and then cease to call it divine."*
>
> *—Hippocrates*

The epilepsy drugs are complicated to use. An effective dose may be only slightly different from an ineffective dose or one that causes intolerable side effects. The drugs have long half-lives[17] and tend to gradually build up in the body until they reach steady state. All of these facts lead to the inescapable truth that prescriptions for medicines to prevent seizures must be compulsively followed.

Human nature encourages patients without symptoms to be inconsistent in their medication compliance. Patients with epilepsy are no exception. If they become seizure-free, they are tempted to stop the medications or lower the dosage without discussion with their physician.

It is possible, of course, that a medication-induced, seizure-free state can be the harbinger of a permanent remission and that medication cessation may be appropriate. However, it is critically important to safely and gradually taper the epilepsy medications, because suddenly stopping a seizure medication can be more dangerous than to have never started it in the first place.

Seizure medications suppress abnormal brain electrical discharges. If this type of medication is abruptly stopped or inappropriately reduced, a sudden increase in brain irritability may trigger rebound seizures and can even lead to life-threatening status epilepticus.[18]

---

[17] A drug half-life is the time needed for half of the medicine to be eliminated or metabolized by the body.

[18] Status epilepticus is a life-threatening condition that occurs when a patient suffers from continuous seizures, or when one seizure follows another in rapid succession without the patient regaining consciousness between seizures.

Summary

Good healthcare requires a meaningful physician-patient partnership. Physicians can fix some conditions, like a surgeon removing an infected appendix or excising a benign brain tumor. However, many of my patients have suffered from chronic conditions that are complex and without known cures. To guide the medical treatment of such long-term afflictions requires that the physician enlist significant patient participation to achieve the best possible outcomes.

People can choose how they live and function despite having life-altering chronic neurological illnesses. These lifestyle choices are not formulas to cure Alzheimer's Disease, headaches, Multiple Sclerosis, Parkinson's Disease, or epilepsy. Yet, increasing evidence shows that wise choices concerning diet, education, and exercise contribute to improved functioning in people afflicted by these maladies.

Epilepsy is used in this chapter as an example to highlight the importance of patient compliance with a proven regimen of medications. Noncompliance is a major factor in breakthrough seizures that can lead to disability, decreased productiveness, or even death.

Widespread variability exists for each individual physician's commitment to patient education and counseling. Even when well educated, patients' ability and/or willingness to successfully embrace a new and healthy lifestyle plan is not assured. As one of my patients put it: "I do really love you doctor. I'm sure you mean well and your recommendations would be helpful. I'm just not sure that I can follow your advice."

Part 2

BECOMING A PHYSICIAN

My career as a neurologist has been long and rewarding, enriched by teaching students and medical residents. My patients enjoyed these young, dedicated individuals, and commonly asked about them when they were absent. Even though I have now retired from the active practice of neurology, my passion for being a physician who specializes in the nervous system persists. My enthusiasm continues unabated to teach and mentor undergraduates, medical students, and residents.

It is easy for me to tell students and medical residents that I have no regrets. I am pleased to have taken the Hippocratic Oath and have spent my career trying to honor the physician-patient social contract it elucidates so clearly. **Chapter 6** reviews my personal medical training and teaching philosophies that developed over time.

As my teaching philosophies matured, it became clear to me that the teaching of medicine and training of physicians relies on the ability to communicate the fundamentals of medical knowledge and the key principles needed for the long-term practice of medicine. **Chapters 7 and 8** encompass an analysis of successful physician practice principles. While everyone would agree that the social-emotional mindfulness principles detailed in **Chapter 8** are obviously of critical importance to a clinician, they are rarely taught or even discussed in most medical training programs.

Chapter 6

The Making of a Physician

The successful transition from a student to an accomplished physician is a complicated process. This transformation is more nuanced than reading and memorizing an enormous body of information, although that is required. As a typical medical student in 1968, I attended hundreds of lectures, participated in multiple lab sessions, and read thousands of pages of text. The journey from student to physician cannot be restricted to gaining insights through laboratory experiments, attending lectures, practicing surgical techniques in the dog labs[19], reading volumes of books and journals, and achieving excellent test scores.

Besides the acquisition and mastery of a voluminous body of information, the education of a clinician includes the development of judgment, honing the skills of listening and communication, remaining empathetic, and always being conscious of treating people with medical conditions, not diseases.

Being a physician is a difficult job, especially when it deals with life and death decisions. For example, what should be done with the 24-year-old woman with the massive stroke? Should she be allowed to die, knowing that she will never again be normal? Should invasive neurosurgery be done without delay to preserve her life, hoping she can enjoy and prosper despite the amount of brain damage she will live with forever?

[19] The "dog labs" are where surgical skills are perfected before operating on people.

> *"To really know is science; to merely believe you know is ignorance."*
> *—Hippocrates*

A physician must have a clear understanding that he is a "professional guesser," without handicapping his ability to be effective if he is not invariably correct. He must be compassionate and humane, yet be able to go on to the next "case" without burdening himself and his family with emotional fallout from caring for the dead and the dying. He must get joy and fulfillment from the practice of medicine and be grateful for the opportunity to practice his profession with humility, grace, and kindness. He must be forever curious and continue as a lifelong learner, who can admit when he does not know something.

Principles of Learning Medicine

The transformation of a physician from a medical student requires the acquisition and implementation of a diverse skill set. A physician must have a unique blend of confidence and self-doubt, decisiveness, and caution. There must also be passion mixed within the functional ability to use "cold" scientific facts untinged by emotional prejudice.

Physicians "practice" medicine. The clinical practice of being a physician entails meaningful dialogue and communication with each patient. It entails the application of medical principles to each individual patient's specific and unique situation.

Good medical schools continually revise their curriculum. At the University of Minnesota, an ongoing dialogue takes place between the basic science professors and the clinicians, seeking to increase the clinical relevance of the basic science courses and infuse the clinical courses with a solid foundation of basic science.

In 2016, the University of Texas at Austin opened the Dell Medical School, which promised to focus its education on healthcare values and collaborative learning methods. This experimental model examines medicine from the point of view of what is best for patients, rather than being organized through the classical silos of surgery, medicine, pediatrics, obstetrics, and psychiatry.

The first Dean of Healthcare Value in America, Dell Medical School's Dr. Christopher Moriates, emphasizes that clinical correlations will be introduced early in the curriculum, while maintaining the primary focus on patient outcomes rather than the medical delivery teams (Clark, 2016b).

The Dell Medical School is the 145th medical school in the country. Our need to train more physicians is accelerating with our aging population and the wide diversity of medical fields and specialties that now exist. Interestingly, Dell is the only school receiving a significant share of its funds from local property taxpayers after a 2012 referendum was approved by 55% of the county. "The community supports being healthy," said Dr. Susan Cox, Dell Medical School's Executive Vice Dean of Academics, "and the idea to create a model healthy community with the medical school at the helm is what got people to vote yes" (Clark, 2016b).

Patient Dialogue and Communication

> ***"It is more important to know the person who has the condition than it is to know the condition the person has."***
> ***—Hippocrates***

A clinician must avoid ego traps, accept responsibility for errors, be careful not to skip key diagnostic steps, and maintain a healthy vigilance as to the diagnosis. In addition, a key to practicing the highest quality medicine is the emphasis on meaningful dialogue and communication with patients and their families. While this sounds obvious, as time pressures increase and medicine continues its drift toward a more impersonal system of care, the primacy of dialogue and communication seems to be eroding, along with the skills to forge meaningful relationships. We must guard against losing these essential skills. **We must focus on caring for *patients*, not *cases*.**

Recent data suggests that "current interns spend the majority of their time in activities only indirectly related to patient care," with less than 15% of the workday spent with their patients. This averages about eight minutes per patient per day with almost half of each day now spent in front of a computer screen. When we consider that "medicine is such an experiential learning experience . . . it's really astonishing that so little time is spent at the patient's bedside" (Chen, 2013).

With these shifts in focus, studies have shown that patient satisfaction is diminishing, outcomes are suffering, and inappropriate prescribing is increasing. Fears are emerging that today's young physicians are likely developing bad habits. With such limited patient interaction, the physicians we are training today may be unable to "recognize the more subtle signs and symptoms of disease or of impending emergencies when they begin practicing on their own" (Chen, 2013).

To rush through "cases" will inevitably lead to a stagnation of the continual process of physician self-improvement and inferior medical care. As Dr. Kathlyn E. Fletcher, Professor of Medicine at the Medical College of Wisconsin in Milwaukee, Wisconsin, said, "There is just no substitute for time spent in doctor-patient relationships. Efficiency is important but it isn't the end of the story" (Chen, 2013).

Learning from Patients

Students spend the first two years in medical school primarily reading, attending lectures, taking tests, and participating in laboratory experiments. Consequently, a third-year medical student in the hospital wards or clinics for the first time is often anxious, confused, and lacking confidence. This was my state of mind when, as a new third-year medical student in the University of Minnesota Hospital, I discovered one of our patients crying in bed. I sat down with the woman to talk. Being hospitalized for almost a week, she was distraught because she felt that nothing was being done and she had not improved.

Her feelings were diametrically opposed to my understanding of her case. My medical team had diagnosed Grave's Disease, a common cause of an overactive thyroid gland known as hyperthyroidism. She had been started on radioactive iodine treatments that would, within a month, begin to correct the overproduction of thyroid hormone and return her to good health. While sitting with her, I explained her diagnosis and our treatment plan.

As she sobbed, it became clear to me that she did not understand all that "medical talk." The primary reason she came to the hospital was diarrhea, a common symptom of hyperthyroidism, which had not improved. As far as she understood, she was not any better. Even as a brand new, third-year medical student, I knew how to order a medicine to relieve her diarrhea. The next day, she was smiling and we were the best of friends. I learned a great deal that day as a neophyte medical student. I learned that listening to patients and engaging them in dialogue is tremendously important. I learned that physicians should talk to patients in language they understand. I learned that physicians should not lecture patients without asking them their thoughts. I learned that the medical staff should educate their patients, not just order tests and treatment. I learned that even the most inexperienced person on a medical team can have a beneficial role by carefully listening.

> ***"The chief virtue language can have is clarity."***
> ***—Hippocrates***

I vividly recall another key experiential learning situation as a senior medical student on the oncology service. My team admitted a cancer patient with a one-month history of a withered right arm. Fortunately, his cancer seemed to be in remission. We peppered the man with questions and performed numerous diagnostic tests, yet, no diagnosis was forthcoming as to why his arm was malfunctioning. We requested consults from other specialties, leading to more tests and arcane theories, without clarifying the cause of the man's problem.

A few days later, I presented the case to Dr. B. J. Kennedy, Chief of the Variety Cancer Center at the University of Minnesota. Dr. Kennedy listened respectfully to my summary of our exhaustive, yet unrevealing workup. As he was familiar with the man from previous admissions, Dr. Kennedy chatted and joked with the man before asking an open-ended question, "How are you doing?"

The man responded that, about a month previously, one of his intravenous chemotherapy infusions had infiltrated into his right arm. Since that complication, his arm had become progressively weaker, atrophic,[20] and almost useless. Forty-five years later, I still remember how foolish it felt to have not calmly allowed the patient to tell his full story in his own words, at his own pace, in his own way. The time lost, the unnecessary tests performed, and the money spent on the patient were lamentable. Fortunately, we had not delayed initiation of any appropriate treatment for the arm weakness, as there was none. However, great caution was recommended during future chemotherapy infusions.

> ***"Life is short, science is long; opportunity is elusive, experiment is dangerous, judgment is difficult."***
> ***—Hippocrates***

---

[20] Atrophic means the wasting away or decrease in the size of an organ or tissue in the body, usually leading to weakness if the affected body part is muscle.

Learning from Fellow Students, Mentors, and Teachers

Medical schools use the team "approach" to provide the best care possible and to advance the knowledge of each team member. I learned a great deal from more experienced team members during my medical internship, followed by my neurology residency.

I was fortunate to be selected in training programs enriched with staff and senior physicians who were eager to teach and good at it. I also learned a great deal by watching. I watched how the other interns, residents, junior staff, and senior staff approached complicated problems and practiced medicine. I watched how they interacted with patients, their families, and the rest of the hospital staff.

Many of the best learning opportunities occur randomly and somewhat unpredictably during "experiential learning" situations, guided by effective tutelage of charismatic and experienced clinicians. There is no effective substitute for a system based on mentoring. Students and physicians in training must be open at any time, day or night, to seize the moment and learn, following the age-old medical wards paradigm: "See one, do one, teach one."

Learning in Medical School

For decades, medical students were ranked on every test, in every class, and at the end of every year. During our first year, the medical school instituted a modified "pass-fail" system. Instead of an "F," the school handed out an "incomplete," requiring that the status change to a "pass" to graduate. Instead of being ranked high, a student who performed above and beyond the requirements of a class was rewarded with the letter grade "O" for "outstanding," while everyone else in each class received a "pass."

No longer focused on class rank, my fellow medical students and I placed primacy on the "big picture," striving to grasp what was clinically relevant, while not "sweating the small stuff."

As previously mentioned, one of our medical students had served as a medic in Vietnam. He encouraged us not to fret when memorizing the names of various blood vessels. "I promise you," he advised, "if a vessel is bleeding, you will tie it off, no matter its name." He reassured us that the clinically relevant anatomy in "the field" or at the time of surgery was not the anatomy taught by the PhD anatomy professors, who were basic scientists and not clinicians. The professors taught what they knew, irrespective of its relevance to the practice of medicine.

A few friends and I developed the enjoyable habit of playing the card game Bridge in the medical student lounge. The card playing even took the place of last-minute, anxious cramming for exams. This relaxed us, allowing better test performance. Other students, who depended on studying at the last minute, were spooked by our card playing, and became discouraged by our confident and calm approach. We were trying to prepare ourselves for a long career in medicine, rather than focusing on stuffing as much information as possible into our brains for a test, irrespective of its importance to our futures.

I loved medical school, especially being full-time in the hospital and clinics during the third and fourth years when the experiential learning began in earnest. Learning on the wards crystallized the establishment of a framework on which to incorporate useful and essential medical information, which was needed for the long term.

Early in the third year, a pediatric resident taught me to respectfully introduce myself to each member of the healthcare team with a smile. He taught me to befriend everyone working in the hospital, emphasizing each person's importance no matter how seemingly menial. It has been my *modus operandi* ever since to have brief, yet meaningful interactions with nursing assistants, dieticians, housekeepers, doormen, transcriptionists, receptionists, housekeepers, secretaries, hospital unit coordinators, and even parking valets. Unfortunately, many of my colleagues treat these workers as if they are invisible.

Neurology residency: I was extremely fortunate to have spent three years as a neurology resident at the University of Minnesota, one of the top training programs in the world in the mid-1970s. This followed a wonderful growth year as a medical intern at Harbor General Hospital in Torrance, California. Harbor General Hospital was an outstanding county hospital and an integral part of the UCLA Medical School teaching system.

Dr. A. B. Baker, our Neurology Department Chairman at the University of Minnesota, was a remarkable clinician and educator. I loved watching him interact with patients, students, and staff. He was a legend, being a founder and the first president of the American Academy of Neurology, which is still headquartered in the Twin Cities. He published the first edition of his definitive, widely distributed textbook, *Clinical Neurology,* in 1955.

Besides leading teaching rounds on the hospital wards, Dr. Baker regularly spent time conducting educational sessions, during which he could masterfully simplify, clarify, and organize the complex body of information constituting the disciplines of neuroanatomy, neurophysiology, and neurochemistry. He and his senior staff were masters at applying the seemingly arcane scientific principles governing the nervous system to practical, everyday patient concerns, thereby setting the teaching standards for neurology in the country and the world.

For the medical students, he published the paperback book called *An Outline of Clinical Neurology* in 1958. For me, this was and still is a 250-page Bible-like tome. It is brief, yet comprehensive and informative. It identifies the overarching principles of diagnosis that apply to all fields of medicine by organizing the vast array of illnesses into five pathological processes: vascular disease, toxic conditions, infections, tumors, and degenerative conditions. In the 21st century, other categories could arguably be added, including autoimmune processes and immunodeficiency disorders.

The *Outline* then focuses on the key elements of the neurological physical examination to localize where the patient's illness likely resides in the nervous system. When combined with the pertinent history, localizing where the problem is in the nervous system is the key to making a correct diagnosis. After all, the nervous system resides everywhere in the body. In addition, while many medical textbooks exclusively emphasized comprehensive differential diagnoses lists, the *Outline* was careful to highlight which diagnoses were common and which were not.

Despite the high-quality didactic sessions, most teaching in residency programs takes place on the hospital wards and clinics, where the science and art of practicing medicine coalesce. Dr. Baker made brilliant diagnoses. He seemed to be able to read people's minds. He treated patients with neurological maladies and patients who feared they had such diseases, using both medical and psychiatric treatment principles as needed.

When appropriate, he used the placebo effect as a powerful tool, and routinely stressed the mind-body connection when traditional medicine and surgery fell short. I watched in amazement as Dr. Baker would cure hysterical paralysis with a placebo device that gave a seemingly useless limb a series of small electrical shocks. With correct patient preparation, this "treatment" approach rarely failed to restore function to a seemingly impaired limb.

Dr. Baker encouraged his neurology residents to be physicians first and specialists second. "Otherwise," he would say, "you will be relegated to the level of a technician." During my residency, we were taught to take care of the entire patient, not just the diagnostic and therapeutic "piece." For example, Dr. Baker's residents were required to know if a patient's home had stairs that would make use of a wheelchair problematic. The residents were expected to consider whether a patient's newly acquired walker would fit into the home bathroom.

Unfortunately, it is common in medicine today for specialists to deal only with diagnostic and therapeutic issues, not the person as a whole. Although physicians still have the ultimate responsibility for the patient, numerous therapists and other professionals are now required to address many of Dr. Baker's concerns.

In our complex fragmented system, "pieces" of the patient are addressed by many specialties, including alternative medicine, palliative care, hospice care, intensive care, social work, and nutritional services. If rehabilitation is needed, the physical medicine and rehabilitation team takes charge, including physiatrists,[21] physical therapists, occupational therapists, speech and language therapists, art therapists, recreational therapists, and mental health therapists.

The University of Minnesota Department of Neurology allowed and encouraged me to serve three months of my residency overseas in London. Dr. Roger Gilliatt, the Chairman of Neurology at the University of London's Neurological Institute at Queen's Square, was my sponsor. Besides being neurologist to the Queen, a renowned researcher in neuromuscular disorders, and an excellent clinician, he was an impressive teacher. Seeing medicine practiced in another country with a different system of medicine was memorable, fascinating, and instructive. This experience expanded my view of clinical medicine, enabling me to consider alternative diagnostic and treatment options during my career.

[21] A physiatrist is a Physical Medicine and Rehabilitation (PM&R) physician.

Being "On Call"

Being "on call" is a somewhat unique part of being trained as a physician. The on-call time is often when a student or a physician in training will have the most responsibility, allowing excellent learning opportunities to gain experience. To be a maximally beneficial learning experience, the opportunity to embrace responsibility must be coupled with appropriate oversight.

When a friend and I were investigating medical internships, we toured a large, sprawling county hospital on the west coast, led by an intern from Minnesota. His year of internship was busy, with extensive periods of on-call autonomy. He explained that he had "seen almost every disease, done every procedure, and prescribed every conceivable treatment" with an enormous amount of independence. While he initially appeared supremely confident, he eventually confided that limited oversight had robbed him of the certainty as to the validity of his treatment choices. My friend and I chose not to apply to that internship.

Being on call eventually becomes a more onerous part of being a physician. It leads to long hours of work with little rest. It leads to unpredictable, rapid-fire crisis management with simultaneous and multiple demands for the physician's attention. I have joked that I wonder how many degrees of separation (interruptions) a physician on call could reasonably be expected to handle, and yet successfully return to and adequately complete the original task in a timely fashion.

For example, in the middle of a hospital consultation, I may be paged by the emergency room to see a possible stroke patient. While talking with the emergency room, a nurse may come up and ask about a different hospitalized patient. While talking to the nurse, my pager may go off, requesting I contact a clinic patient, then his pharmacy. While on the phone with the pharmacy, I may be notified of an urgent ICU consult of a patient who just lapsed into unresponsiveness. Hopefully, the original hospitalized patient I had been interviewing would understand the significance of the urgent matters that took me from his bedside and my juggling of these disparate issues would not adversely affect his care.

The ability to be on call and calmly, intelligently prioritize the importance of multiple divergent issues is a key physician skill that must be acquired. This skill is rarely discussed, let alone "taught" to medical students. It is common knowledge that the interaction that triggers an angry "blow up" or "meltdown" is often caused by the circumstances that preceded the over-reaction. Certainly, an on-call doctor stressed by multi-tasking is a classic setup for a "blow up." Hopefully, our training programs are beginning to address the advantages and perils of the physician on-call model and educate the physicians appropriately.

Please understand that being on call can invoke some of the most rewarding experiences in the professional life of a physician. As one of my senior partners, Dr. Richard Foreman, often reminded me, the patients and their families are often very appreciative of the availability of a physician coming to their aid late at night or on a weekend.

Time Management

Time management is a challenging issue for a physician. It is, of course, frustrating for a patient to wait in a doctor's office. Rarely is it known if the next clinic or hospital patient will be a routine matter or a complex crisis that demands additional time. The staff rarely knows in advance the complexity of the required physician-patient encounter or the appropriate time to be allotted.

Unfortunately, a patient of mine was kept waiting for over two hours in the clinic one day. When I finally entered his exam room, he smiled and calmly remarked, "Thank you for seeing me now." I was speechless after this unexpected sentiment of appreciation until he laughed and continued, "I was almost fossilized in the waiting room, doc."

My schedule was continually in flux. Fortunately, my practice at Neurological Associates of St. Paul was blessed with a wonderful, knowledgeable, and helpful staff to help cope when the physician's schedules disintegrated under the pressure of caring for those who needed immediate assistance.

Nonetheless, predicting the time needed to address a clinic patient's needs is difficult. For example, patients with headaches are commonly seen in neurological offices, yet their diagnoses and assessment requirements may be dramatically dissimilar:

- A new headache patient may only require a standard 30-45 minute consultation, while another new headache patient may have a life-threatening problem that needs extended time.

- A headache patient may have seen numerous doctors and arrive with a long and complex history of testing and unsuccessful treatment regimens. This patient will benefit from a prolonged discussion of a complicated, multifaceted treatment approach to the chronic headaches.
- A patient's syndrome might be a benign muscle tension phenomenon requiring only brief patient reassurance.
- A patient with a benign muscle tension headache syndrome, however, may require a prolonged discussion of lifestyle changes and complex medication adjustments.
- A patient may be diagnosed as having classic migraine headaches that will require an intermediate amount of time to prescribe a new prescription and a homework assignment of educational reading.

Stroke patients who come to the clinic for a follow-up may also have disparate needs:

- If a recently discharged stroke victim recovered with no other concerns, the patient might reasonably be scheduled for a 15-minute follow-up visit.
- A high-risk stroke patient may require a complex and prolonged visit to address the risk factors to prevent another occurrence.
- Another patient might require additional stroke education, continuing therapy, or a review of the medication requirements and compliance.
- Occasionally, it might be prudent to reassess a patient for the possibility of a new stroke, medical complications, or other complicating medical issues.

Hospital encounters also vary considerably in complexity and time required. Many times over the years, as I prepared to leave the hospital on the way to the clinic, an emergency arose, demanding my immediate attention and delaying my arrival at the office. During our second year of marriage, my wife and I lived in Los Angeles during my internship. My wonderfully understanding wife identified two rules that seemed to govern the unpredictable length of my daily hospital shifts:

- The longer the intern was in the hospital, the longer the intern was in the hospital.
- The more patients the intern had, the more patients the intern had.

Over the years, I commonly ran late in the clinic, sometimes necessitating long waiting times for my patients. Fortunately, I have been blessed overall with understanding patients. When running late, I have learned not to hurry patients, instead treating each person as an important individual with a significant medical concern. No matter the wait, patients understood that when their time came to see me, they would have my complete and undivided attention without being rushed.

Learning from Other Practitioners and Staff

> ***"The life so short, the craft so long to learn."***
> ***—Hippocrates***

My learning from other physicians did not end after my graduation from the neurology residency. Many experienced community physicians took me under their wing, giving me encouragement and words of wisdom. I eagerly listened to and loved their stories.

Many years ago, a senior family practitioner overheard me talking about a "good case" of a patient with an unusual malignant brain tumor. "Paul," he said, "an unusual, malignant brain tumor that will cause the patient to die is not what I would call a 'good case.'" He went on to humorously describe a "good case" as "a patient that comes to the office with a tension headache that is alleviated by giving him a couple of pills. He then happily pays the office bill on the way out." Besides being an excellent clinician, this physician was a practical and compassionate man.

Another remarkable general practitioner (GP)[22] stressed the use of common sense when recommending treatment. A family brought a severely demented Alzheimer's patient to him for a second opinion. An ophthalmologist had recommended that the patient have her cataracts removed. The GP thought for a moment, frowned, then opined that it was unnecessary to put the elderly woman through the eye surgery. He told the family that "to take out her cataracts would be like changing the lens in a camera with no film in it."

Early in my career, a highly regarded internist told me matter-of-factly: "You will

---

[22] General practitioners (GP) entered the practice of primary care medicine directly after an internship; they have now been replaced by Family Physicians (FP), who enter the practice of medicine only after satisfactorily completing at least a three-year medical residency.

not be liked by every patient, because of their different personalities and expectations. You must be yourself." For example some patients:

- Want the truth and some do not.
- Have realistic expectations and some do not.
- Come prepared to give a complete history and some do not.
- Will honestly and accurately report their lifestyle, good and bad habits alike, and some will not.
- Are very emotional and some are not.

Patients Pick a Physician

People have varied motivations to see certain physicians. Dr. Terrance Capistrant, one of my senior partners, explained to me early in my career that patients often choose a physician by "quality, cost, and convenience . . . but in the reverse order." Sometimes he put it this way: "Patients choose a physician by ability, affordability, availability, and affability . . . but in the reverse order." In many cases, he explained, patients assume quality care will be delivered.

Patients tend to gravitate to physicians with certain personalities, reputations, and practice styles, which can enhance medical care, although not invariably. To seek out the best trained and most communicative physician is rarely a bad idea. It is not easy, however, to identify the best doctors. Physician lists, such as "Top Doctors," have some validity, although they are imperfect and certainly do not clarify which doctor is right for a specific patient with a specific condition. As of yet, an accurate, meaningful tabulation of "batting averages" for physicians has not been developed.

Besides convenience, cost (with insurance coverage being a huge factor), and bedside manner, some patients choose physicians based on their:

- Willingness to provide narcotics more readily than their peers.
- Ordering enough tests to exceed the "no fault" automobile insurance threshold, allowing a patient to bring a lawsuit more easily.
- History of rarely finding anything wrong with patients involved in litigation, leading insurance companies and defense attorneys to favor them.
- Adherence to national criteria for avoiding unnecessary testing and

treatment options, causing some patients to shun such best practice, yet "minimalist" care.

- Reputation to be conservative or aggressive in their indications for surgery.

In the words of Bob Dylan, "Times they are a-changin." We are now in the era of big data, which promises to improve the public's discernment as to quality medical care. Survival rates, complications, and charges for various conditions and surgeries are being more accurately tracked, tabulated, and recorded. Registries of cancer treatment protocols and outcomes are now common.

Medicare meaningful use data for various practitioners are beginning to be accumulated and likely will be published in some form in the near future. A few states publish yearly reports listing hospital-based errors, such as patient falls and hospital-acquired infections, treatment results, and charges.

Increasing numbers of certified and accredited centers exist for specific diseases, such as stroke. While not a guarantee of excellence, accreditation shows, at a minimum, that the institution is tracking, documenting, and reporting some meaningful quality of care measures.

With medicine embracing the business model, the dramatic growth of social media, the widespread availability of the internet, increasing financial pressures, and new avenues of government intervention, more information is becoming available about physicians, clinics, and hospitals. Patient satisfaction surveys are becoming more popular. Fees and charges are beginning to be published. Even Angie's List[23] has begun evaluating doctors.

Summary

To learn the practice of medicine, a motivated person must study and train for many years to complete an internship, residency, and possibly one or more fellowships. Physicians must attend hundreds of lectures and labs and read thousands of medical articles and scores of books. However, a critical key in the development of a skillful physician is "on-the-job" training to gain knowledge, judgment, and wisdom.

---

[23] Angie's List is a common rating and review list for service providers.

This involves:

- Watching and listening to skillful mentors.
- Experiential learning: Hands-on learning by doing, with appropriate oversight.
- Listening to the patients and their families, to other members of the medical team, and to one's colleagues and associates.
- Developing realistic self-confidence while maintaining humility and empathy.
- Mastering the art of in-depth, personal communication.
- Acknowledging the value of each member of the medical team.
- Practicing time management skills while accepting the unpredictability in medicine.
- Mastering teaching and oversight of others on the medical team.
- Being aware of stress, while developing enhanced coping mechanisms.
- Lifelong learning.

The training of a physician is a long, arduous process. To enter medicine, a student must realize that mastering this profession is not equivalent to running a sprint. Mastering medicine is akin to entering a marathon with no finish line until retirement.

Chapter 7

Physician Practice Principles: The Knowledge Needed to Practice Medicine

During my 45 years of being in medicine, I have learned important lessons in how a physician practices medicine. In medicine, as in life, to learn is one thing, but to understand what is learned is quite another thing. A typical physician has learned millions of facts over years and years of study. To meaningfully apply these facts, when appropriate, is the true physician skill.

It is now clear that human beings possess multiple intelligences (Gardner, 1993). An enhanced level of each enables a physician to provide excellent patient care over the long term. Physician practice principles encompass dynamic, unique, yet overlapping skills and knowledge sets. It is my contention that these fundamental physician skill sets include:

- Intellectual acquisition and application of medical knowledge.
- Lifelong curiosity.
- Social-emotional mindfulness.

No physician can succeed without the ability to possess and utilize the enormous body of medical knowledge, focusing primarily on prevention, evaluation, and treatment of illness. Many clinicians, especially neurologists, are accused of being compulsively organized, detail-focused, and nerdy in their quest to make a positive difference in their patient's lives. Neurologists are indeed typically compulsive and their attention to detail is legendary.

All clinicians must master the skills of history taking, performing an excellent physical exam, and formulating a comprehensive differential diagnosis [24] and proper treatment plan. Like other physicians, a neurologist should be intelligently decisive, yet humble enough to periodically reevaluate her diagnoses and treatment plans.

Most physicians no longer practice in isolation, as a rare hospitalized patient sees only one physician, while many clinic patients are also referred to specialists from time to time. Physicians must master the art of communication, not just with patients, but also with colleagues. Neurologists, often serving as a consultant, must craft detailed, useful reports. In addition, a successful physician must adjust to the evolving role and accurate interpretation of medical testing, learn to effectively relieve pain and suffering, pursue lifelong education, and, in my case, continue a lifelong commitment to teaching.

Intellectual Acquisition and Application of Medical Knowledge

The first requirement to successfully become a physician is the acquisition of information. No physician can succeed without the ability to possess and utilize a large body of facts.

Learning techniques: The acquisition of enormous amounts of information does not guarantee success as a clinician. Among the important skills that must be perfected to thrive as a clinician is the mastery of various learning techniques. To best learn the practice of medicine, I have found it most efficacious to master three or four fundamental features of each disease, medication, and subject, which I refer to as "bedrock" information. Having mastered the bedrock information in each instance allows for the natural upgrade and incremental expansion of knowledge as needed during the evolution of an individual practitioner's practice of medicine.

This approach favors the "lumpers over the splitters." "Lumpers" tend to coalesce information into recognizable groups with commonalities, while "splitters"

[24] A differential diagnosis is a list of diagnostic possibilities, which hopefully incorporates the final, correct diagnosis.

typically gain knowledge by identifying differences among various conditions and/or treatments.

This approach is in contrast to the common student approach of memorizing everything possible for a test, rarely discriminating the importance of numerous nuggets of information. Reliance on memorization and regurgitation at test time is actually the educational norm prior to medical school clinical rotations. This approach suffers from the unfortunate tendency of having a random exponential decay curve for the facts memorized, irrespective of the future needs of the student.

Some students, therefore, have difficulty transitioning from studying for "the test" to mastering what is of long-term importance. Yet, success in the emergency room, the wards, and the clinics demands immediate access to a fundamentally sound knowledge base (what I referred to above as "bedrock knowledge") that can be expanded and deepened as the situation demands.

Most fields of clinical medicine, like neurology, are challenging in so far as they require the mastery of the complex disciplines of anatomy, biochemistry, and physiology, superimposed upon excellent "people skills." All of this basic science information, when combined with advanced clinical skills, is then utilized to diagnose, treat, educate, and counsel patients.

Tenets of good clinical medical education: I believe three important tenets are necessary in the successful education of medical residents and students. A good teacher is the first tenet, although individuals require varying degrees of guidance and mentoring.

Second, material from which to learn is obviously of crucial importance in clinical medicine, as vast amounts of information must be analyzed and acquired. The material is available in books, literature searches, and didactic lectures. It is acquired in discussions with colleagues and other experts. In large part, clinical medicine must be learned "at the bedside," which means widespread exposure to appropriate patients is essential.

Third, students and medical residents require a sufficient amount of responsibility to learn judgment and decision-making skills, best accomplished with appropriate oversight. While much can be learned through passive observation, judgment is best acquired by doing. No substitute exists for having actual responsibility to perform a patient interview and examination, make a diagnosis, and formulate a diagnostic and therapeutic plan.

To effectively utilize opportunities for patient responsibility, the student must assume that he will make a difference in the patient's life. It has been said: "A good physician in training must get his hands dirty; he must lose both his fear and his lack of grace to succeed."

As the least trained, least knowledgeable, and least experienced medical team member, the student who hopes to make a difference must be the most conscientiously thorough team member. His patient evaluation and interviews must be the most complete. He must do all the little things. He must go the extra mile to research appropriate diagnostic and therapeutic issues, while attempting to formulate independent conclusions. By necessity, the senior staff in a successful teaching program must have the final word as astute clinical judgment rarely develops overnight.

Taking the patient history: The first step in a clinical evaluation of a person with a medical problem is taking the patient's history. This begins immediately, even before words are spoken. It begins with the first glance at a patient's name and age. Physically, it begins with the handshake. Physicians should introduce themselves and attempt to correctly pronounce the patient's name. Unfortunately, physicians do not always introduce themselves.

In her book *Visual Intelligence* (2016), Amy E. Herman highlights a medical student's unique understanding of the physician-patient interaction:

> I never thought of myself as a translator, but that's essentially what we're all doing when we communicate effectively; we're translating our message to one another. When I see patients, they describe their complaints and concerns to me subjectively because it's about how they're feeling. I then translate that into objective symptoms that can be treated. However, if I speak to them from my own reference point, they might not understand. In fact, the medical terminology generally confuses or alarms people. I have to translate my own message of diagnosis into something that's easily understood from their perspective (p. 188).

While formulating an approach to the patient's medical problem, the physician should resist the temptation to prematurely place her patient's case into a narrow diagnostic cubbyhole. It is good medical practice to let the patient talk. It is good medical practice to listen. It is good medical practice to say, "What else?" repeatedly throughout the patient's recitation of the history until the patient has thoughtfully and thoroughly finished his story. In my experience, "What else?" serves as a better invitation for the patient to raise other issues than "Anything else?"

A patient encounter is, in large part, a healthcare investigative process. These "what else?" questions employed by physicians to clarify a patient's problem can be considered a doctor's corollary to the "Five Whys" of Toyota Production (Ohno, 2006). Toyota's "Five Whys" serve as an in-depth exploration of the cause-and-effect relationship underlying a particular production problem. This system repeatedly asks "why," delving deeper and deeper until the root cause of the problem becomes crystallized. As in the search for production efficiency, by asking, "What else?" a physician creates an environment wherein all pertinent issues are identified early.

A reasonable and usable approach to interviewing patients includes establishing a connection with the patient (building rapport), expressing empathy, formulating a plan that is clear to the patient, and allowing time to answer all the patient's questions. While these steps seem obvious, they can be overshadowed by a complicated medical condition. Physicians must remember, especially in complicated situations, that a complete patient history may require interviewing family members, friends, and caregivers. Especially in patients with cognitive impairment, the perceptions of people close to the patient may hold valuable information that may not be elicited if only the patient is interviewed.

The diagnostic process can be the equivalent of solving a puzzle. In her search for the answer, a clinician may inappropriately focus on the puzzle rather than on the patient, who in reality is a unique individual with a problem. At times, the arduous and time consuming process of gathering and documenting all the information needed may interfere with the physician's attempt to establish rapport, empathy, and address each of the patient's questions, concerns, and fears. A successful physician rarely lets that occur.

Successfully performing the physical examination: After taking the patient history, a well-performed examination (in my case, the neurological examination) is an undeniably key component in the diagnostic process. As spelled out below, the four-step approach to making a diagnosis is sacrosanct, especially in a neurologist's toolbox. The exam serves the valuable function of identifying where the medical problem resides and the extent of the abnormalities, which typically leads to clarifying the actual diagnosis.

As a first-year medical student, I was sent to examine a sick man and emerged with no clue as to his illness. I struggled mightily for an hour at the bedside with the multiple small tasks encompassed in a complete physical exam. Everything was new to me, including the exam of his eyes, ears, heart, lungs, abdomen, pelvis, muscular strength, and the deep tendon reflexes.

After summarizing my evaluation to my instructor and admitting I was clueless as to the diagnosis, I introduced my instructor to the patient. From the doorway, my instructor turned to me and asked that I look at the man. When I looked at the man as a person rather than focusing on the pieces of the exam, I was shocked and embarrassed that I had not observed he was visibly yellow, suggesting he was jaundiced from a liver disease like hepatitis.

The physical exam incorporates multiple, important mechanical tasks, yet in its entirety, it includes observational talents that must be cultivated. This remains true even in today's hurried, technologically focused delivery system. In Amy E. Herman's words, "Students need to realize that no matter how helpful technology has become, it is no match [for] a good set of eyes and a brain" (2016, p. 19).

In addition, the successful clinician is careful to conscientiously and independently evaluate each patient. As Herman warns:

> In the managed-healthcare world, where monetary rewards are given for seeing as many patients as quickly as possible, the medical professionals can be tempted to sacrifice quality care for quantity care and go straight for the patient's chart in an effort to expedite the visit, relying on what the caregiver before them has written before personally evaluating a patient and making observations of their own (2016, p. 17).

The scope and diversity of human disease demands that different examinations are needed in various situations. The neurologist, for example, must tailor the exam to the needs of the individual patient. Patients suffering from memory loss, stroke, seizure, coma, herniated disc, spinal cord disorder, or peripheral nerve maladies require unique examination approaches. For a patient with cognitive complaints, a thorough cognitive assessment alone may require one to two hours to complete.

The physician must use judgment in determining when to delve more deeply into specific elements of the exam. **Judgment comes from experience; experience comes from practice.**

Professor Dr. Roger Gilliatt, my mentor at University of London's Neurological Institute at Queen's Square, emphasized that the neurological exam was not to look "at things," but was most productive when it was used to look "for things." In essence, he preached that a successful physical examination was best accomplished when the neurologist knows what she is looking for, rather than doing the identical standardized exam for each person, no matter the medical problem.

Four-step sacrosanct approach to making a diagnosis: Beginning with the history and continuing through the examination and testing, physicians (especially neurologists) do their best work when they follow a four-step diagnostic process:

Step 1: Clarify the onset of the problem: It is of crucial importance to establish exactly what the situation was when the problem began. Define whether the illness began suddenly (like a heart attack or stroke), subacutely (like an infection), or gradually (like a tumor or a degenerative process).

Step 2: Document the course of the illness from the beginning to the present time: Has the disease been worsening or improving since the onset? Has the medical malady been stable or fluctuating? Each of these courses typically leads the physician to consider a different group of diseases.

Step 3: Localize the lesion[25]: Where is the nidus[26] of the problem? Although identifying the site of disease is of obvious importance in medicine, in neurology it is of particular significance because the nervous system involves the entire body. The nervous system is divided in two parts: the peripheral nervous system (PNS) and the central nervous system (CNS). The PNS is comprised of the muscles, neuromuscular junction, and peripheral nerves, while the CNS, comprised of the brain and spinal cord, resides quite well protected within the skull and the spinal canal.

Let's consider an example of a patient with a numb big toe. The importance of localizing the lesion becomes clear when we compile a list of the possible sites of disease or injury. These include:

---

[25] Lesion is an injury or disease of a part of the body.

[26] Nidus is a site of origin.

- A local process in the foot (like inflammatory joint disease) involving tiny local nerves.
- A large nerve injury in the leg (like nerve trauma at the knee).
- A dysfunction of the plexus[27] of nerves in the pelvis (like from a tumor).
- Damage to a nerve root in the lower back (like being compressed by a herniated disc).
- A spinal cord process (like Multiple Sclerosis).
- A disease of the brain (like a tumor, blood clot, or stroke).

In other words, by localizing the lesion, the neurologist can avoid investigating and imaging the body from head to foot.

Step 4: Determine the diagnosis or formulate a differential diagnosis: Despite the temptation to "leap" ahead to this final step, it is rarely prudent. Time saved initially by skipping Steps 1, 2, or 3 may lead to inappropriate testing, delayed diagnosis, and wasted time. In the long term, mistakes will more often be made when a physician does not assiduously adhere to this simple four-step diagnostic process.

Common diseases are common: Another key principle in the learning of medicine is to begin by focusing on what's common or likely. It turns out that common diseases are indeed common. Believing that being thorough is paramount, many practitioners, especially the young and inexperienced, may get sidetracked attempting to consider every possibility, no matter how remote. It is well known that more diagnostic possibilities exist in the rare 20% compared to the number of illnesses that make up the common 80%. I refer to this focus on every possibility as a bad case of the "what ifs."

"A physician must learn to recognize the common diseases and the rare ones that have treatments; then the rest of medicine can then be her hobby."
—Unknown

Of course, all successful physicians should be able to identify rare conditions as well as the common ones. Interestingly, a rare disease, being often unique, may be readily identified. An uncommon presentation of a common disease may be the most difficult

[27] A nerve plexus is a branching network of intersecting nerves.

diagnosis of all, as common maladies may have a myriad of ways they present. As we emphasize on teaching rounds, the patients have not read the textbook, so their disease presentation may not be a textbook scenario.

Communicate with other medical providers and craft useful consultation reports: As a neurologist, I have spent my professional life as a consultant communicating with patients and referring physicians. Although this was not emphasized in my training, it quickly became clear that the consultation report must be crafted in a clear and understandable format, ideally organized in three parts. First, the specialist should open with a succinct summary reviewing the facts and theories preceding the consult. Second, the specialist should delineate new facts and/or information currently available. Third, the specialist needs to answer the question that triggered the consult or suggest an appropriate plan to resolve the problem.

Sometimes the consult request asks an obvious question, for example, "What is the diagnosis?" or "What treatment do you recommend?" Sometimes the reason for the consult is less obvious, especially if the diagnosis and treatment plans are clear. The question may be as simple as a request for validation of the existing diagnosis and/or treatment plan. Alternatively, the request may be for the consultant to discuss the prognosis with the family. Therefore, even after a complete and comprehensive assessment, the consultation is unfinished without documenting a family discussion.

Periodically reevaluate the diagnosis, the treatment plan, and the current state of the patient's daily functioning: A significant part of a physician's skill set is the ability to periodically rethink cases, especially if the diagnosis seems forced or if all available facts do not neatly fit into place. With the knowledge that, as humans, we make mistakes, we must be forever vigilant and humble.

I have an aversion to physicians who are too arrogant to reassess an earlier decision. Physicians should not be like a horse wearing blinders meant to decrease distractions and keep the horse on the chosen path. Especially during a complicated case, a physician should periodically review the patient's situation from multiple vantage points to assess whether the medical team is following the best way forward.

For example, a few years ago I re-evaluated a woman's diagnosis of Multiple Sclerosis. She had been treated to prevent MS flare-ups for ten years and had experienced none. At the onset, her symptoms were typical of MS, although her physical examination and testing were more nuanced and subtle. Was the treatment successful or could she possibly not have MS? My skepticism led me to doubt the diagnosis. While safe, her treatment entailed daily, self-administered shots that were expensive, uncomfortable, and inconvenient. After retesting and a discussion, she reluctantly agreed to discontinue the treatment and has fortunately remained disease-free.

Another reason that physicians should periodically re-examine previous decisions is that medical "truths" evolve and change. What was once thought to be true may change. For example, what constitutes a healthy diet is continually being revised. It now seems clear that moderate amounts of red wine, dark chocolate, and eggs may be prudent and healthy.

Re-evaluation of a medical case should also address how the disease currently affects a person's life, day-to-day, week-to-week, and year-to-year. Physicians deal with people who have disease and should focus on their patients' physical well-being and coping skills. Even if the disease progression has slowed, its influence on a patient's life may have changed. As opposed to focusing solely on the characteristics of illness, the importance of intermittently discussing a patient's life, ability to function, and goals cannot be overemphasized.

Effectively and efficiently understanding the role of medical testing: A physician's role includes the use of their knowledge and experience to consider when it is appropriate to do medical testing. This sounds easier than it actually is. Testing must be intelligently and carefully considered. While there are increased efforts today to attempt to discourage the widespread, inappropriate testing (and treatments) because of high costs, complications, and false positives, multiple forces are continuing to drive more testing. Some of these forces include:

1. Patient expectations and demands: Patients and their families are becoming more distrustful of physicians when given a diagnosis without substantiated testing. As previously noted, some individuals believe that testing is the true mark of a thorough medical investigation. It is not uncommon to hear complaints that a doctor did "nothing" when no tests were ordered, despite an accurate diagnosis and appropriate advice being provided after a thorough history and physical assessment.

A clinic patient of mine complained that my consultation fee was too high, as I had "spent only five minutes" with him. Because of this complaint, I called him and read him my consultation report. After hearing my report, he agreed that my consult three months earlier "must have lasted longer than five minutes" for me to have learned all the information spelled out in the dictation. Although I reassured him that "nothing was seriously wrong," he still felt my consult fee was too high and could be in error because no testing was done.

My uncle Morrie saw a neurologist at my suggestion because of the sudden onset of a left-sided facial paralysis. Although he was correctly diagnosed and treated for Bell's Palsy,[28] he complained, "Paul, how could that doctor charge me for a consultation when he did not even have me drop my pants or do tests?"

2. Defensive medical practice: Physicians, at times, justify excessive testing out of fear of malpractice lawsuits. However, most experts agree that lawsuits are minimized when a physician performs a thorough history and examination, is honest with patients, and establishes patient rapport.

Let me recite a not so far-fetched scenario. After a careful history and exam, *physician A* correctly diagnoses migraine without ordering a brain scan. Without testing, the patient remains worried, goes "doctor shopping," and persuades *physician B* to order a brain scan. While the scan is not perfectly normal, it neither detects anything serious or identifies a reason for the patient's headaches, which are indeed migraines. Even though *physician A's* diagnosis was confirmed, the discovery of an abnormality on the testing, although unrelated to the patient's headaches, may trigger the upset and distrustful patient to unnecessarily criticize "sloppy" *physician A*. The patient may even attempt to damage *physician A's* reputation, while raising the possibility of an inappropriate malpractice lawsuit. Who can blame *physician A* for ordering unnecessary brain scans in the future?

A recently published study did lend credence to the hypothesis that more tests may indeed protect a doctor from malpractice cases. This study analyzed 18.3 million Florida hospital discharges from 2000-2009 (Jena, 2015). After adjusting for patient characteristics, comorbidities, and diagnoses, the study found that greater average physician spending on testing was associated with a decreased risk of incurring a malpractice claim.

On the other hand, a different research paper emphasized that over-dependence on imaging testing, associated with less reliance on a detailed patient history and physical, contributes to more diagnostic medical errors (Fallik, 2016b). In addition, medical errors were correlated with doctor bias and the stereotyping of certain

[28] Bell's Palsy is the sudden weakness of one-half of the facial muscles.

patient populations.

3. The process of training physicians often focuses on testing: Although we conscientiously teach medical students to take careful patient histories, as young doctors progress through training programs, more emphasis is placed on specialized testing. As more ingenious tests are developed, residencies and fellowships by necessity spend ever increasing amounts of time to understand and master these tests.

After graduating from advanced specialty training, it is not surprising that these newly minted doctors focus on procedures and testing in clinical practice. Remarkably, I cannot recall one instance of a teaching professor criticizing the on-call neurology resident for doing excessive testing, despite numerous instances of the on-call resident being grilled for not considering alternative diagnoses, which would have led to unnecessary testing.

4. Testing tends to save physicians' time: Busy physicians are often tempted to default to testing rather than embarking on a time-consuming patient interview and careful detailed examination. In addition, when a patient requests an unnecessary test, time may again be a consideration. It is often quicker to order the requested test than to spell out in detail why it is unnecessary.

5. Financial considerations fostered by skewed incentives: Besides the time considerations, direct financial considerations enter into the current practice of medicine. As discussed earlier, it is not a secret that our healthcare system has financial incentives which favor testing and procedures over interviewing and counseling patients.

6. Physician illusion of control: I was fascinated to read an article theorizing the existence of a physician's "illusion of control," with a corollary that a physician's "therapeutic illusion" also exists. This theory suggests that physicians tend to overestimate the benefits of what they do, which is reinforced by a "confirmation bias." When a physician identifies a treatment or testing success, he may inappropriately generalize this effect. To be more objective, the physician should carefully look for contradictory evidence of failure of the treatment or testing in question. Without careful analysis, these unrecognized psychological tendencies likely contribute to over testing and inappropriate treatment recommendations (Casarett, 2016).

Accurately interpreting medical testing results: Besides being ever vigilant to avoid unnecessary testing, a physician must learn to accurately interpret testing results and explain the results to the patients in ways they will understand. For example, one of my patients was confused by a cardiologist who told the patient that "the heart monitoring was normal with some abnormalities." I clarified for her that the infrequent arrhythmia documented on the testing was of no clinical significance and therefore of no concern.

Several years ago, a distinguished university professor confided in me that a modern definition of a normal person might be "someone who has not had a CT of the chest, as most scans have some spot or scar." He was stressing, of course, the importance of having a very good reason to order such a test, knowing that the results commonly trigger angst and require follow-up testing.

Many of today's imaging studies are exquisitely sensitive, leading to many "abnormal results," many of which are insignificant. Neurological consultations are not infrequently triggered by an unexpected abnormality on just such a study. Two representative examples are cerebral aneurysms and spinal degenerative changes.

Cerebral aneurysms: Sometimes testing reveals findings that are indeed fortuitous, such as a large asymptomatic aneurysm, which can be safely repaired before causing a life-threatening crisis. On the other hand, neuroradiologists frequently identify tiny, unruptured, asymptomatic cerebral aneurysms on brain MRI scans. Many of these aneurysms are of no clinical significance, being unlikely to cause a problem other than angst. The availability of a noninvasive, nonsurgical treatment option that secures cerebral aneurysms by placing a coil during a cerebral angiogram has complicated the decision to treat, to watch, or to ignore these tiny aneurysms.

Spinal degenerative changes: The medical literature is quite clear that a patient's symptoms and spinal imaging abnormalities may be dramatically discordant. As opposed to the asymptomatic small cerebral aneurysms discussed above, spinal disc-degenerative disease is typically discovered because of complaints of back or neck pain. Therefore, it may not be clear what should be done, because spinal degenerative disease can and does cause pain. However, surgery is rarely helpful if the options are carefully analyzed and best medical practice guidelines are followed.

Unfortunately, thousands of unnecessary, complicated, expensive, and potentially dangerous spinal surgeries are performed every year in America. While the abnormalities on the imaging studies can be repaired surgically, the emphasis should be on long-term patient disability. In other words, a patient's ability to maintain a healthy level of physical activity is the appropriate goal, not the correction of imaging abnormalities of questionable clinical significance.

Let me be clear, isolated back or neck pain is rarely a valid indication for major spinal surgery. Our spines "wear out" and degenerate over time with resulting pain. Fusing one, two, or three spinal vertebral bodies does not prevent further spinal degeneration and rarely leads to a pain-free existence. It has been shown that the spine above and below the surgical fusions degenerates more quickly. Spinal surgery should not be performed if it does not enhance patient functionality or lead to long-term symptom improvement.

Of course, valid indications for spinal surgery exist, including nerve damage, nerve or spinal cord impingement, identification of infection or tumor, and spinal instability. Even with a clear indication for surgery, the surgery that is performed may often be overly extensive. When operating on a symptomatic spinal lesion, many surgeons will expand the surgery to include asymptomatic lesions seen on imaging studies. This adds expense, while increasing the risk without adding proven benefit.

Spinal stenosis,[29] which causes compression of spinal nerves or spinal cord by a degeneration of the spine, is a valid surgical indication. The simplest surgery to remove the compression of the spinal nerves is a bilateral laminectomy.[30] Many surgeons choose to perform a more complex surgery "just to be sure," fusing the vertebral bodies together instead of simply decompressing the spinal canal. To the patient, a fusion sounds more definitive. The patient rarely understands that it doubles the potential complication rate, delays recovery, increases the cost, and is of minimal additional value (Moon, 2016).

Following complex surgery with a prolonged recovery, it may be difficult for the patient to determine whether the surgery was worth it. In some cases, the patients experience a "flight to health,"[31] strongly influencing their opinion of the surgical result. To some extent, this is a placebo effect. As far as a placebo response is concerned, it is not surprising that the more invasive treatments have the highest

---

[29] Spinal stenosis exists when degeneration of the spine has led to a narrowing of the spinal canal.

[30] Laminectomy is the surgical procedure of removing the back of the vertebral bodies (the lamina) to relieve pressure on the spinal cord or on the nerve roots.

[31] Flight to health occurs when a patient wills himself or herself to feel better after a treatment, whether or not the treatment is useful.

percentage of positive placebo responses. Surgery, including spinal surgery, therefore, has a more potent placebo effect than medication trials or physical therapy.

The financial incentives in medicine encourage complex spinal surgeries despite the absence of definitive proof in many circumstances, especially in patients with isolated back or neck pain. Spinal surgery is very well reimbursed; the more complex the spinal surgery, the higher the reimbursement. Sadly, when surgical complications occur, necessitating repeat surgery, the surgeon, the anesthesiology team, and the hospital are paid again under the prevailing medical reimbursement system. Only the patient suffers.

With the aging of the population, spinal surgery demands will likely increase, with some estimates suggesting a 59% increase by the year 2025 over the current amount of spinal surgery (Dykes & Chase, 2016). Because the demand for surgery, such as spine surgery, has "far outpaced our ability to measure and report effectiveness of the procedures," a need clearly exists for standardized outcome information, including Patient-Reported Outcome data (Dykes & Chase, 2016, p. 34). I am confident that this will occur and shape our practice, hopefully in the relatively near future.

Appropriately relieving pain and suffering: One of the tenets of the Hippocratic Oath is to relieve pain and suffering. However, a crisis in American medicine has developed over the last 20 years, triggering a narcotic epidemic of epic proportions. A newspaper headline in April 2016 screamed, "Opioid Reliance: One of the Great Mistakes in Medical History" (Scott, 2016).

While an important facet of practicing medicine is acquiring the competence to treat pain, this skill acquisition has not been emphasized in many medical training programs. In addition to training shortfalls, the difficulties of dealing with chronic pain patients has led to the development of an independent specialty of pain management. This unfortunate development coincided with a national campaign to treat pain as a vital sign, with a goal of completely eliminating pain whenever possible. While this sounds like a laudable goal, in practice the treatment of pain is more nuanced, complicated, and fraught with the risk of addiction.

A relatively new organization called Physicians for Responsible Opioid Prescribing is asking that pain as a fifth vital sign be amended, and that patient satisfaction questions about chronic pain be removed from the Joint Commission of Hospital Accreditation reimbursement procedures (Fiore, 2016). The treatment of a temporarily painful process, like a herniated disc, broken bone, or trigeminal neuralgia, should be treated aggressively. The treatment of pain from advanced cancer should be managed vigorously and humanely. However, the "war on pain" led to the unconscionable overtreatment of benign and chronic pain when safer and reasonably effective remedies were available. This resulted in addicting thousands of people to narcotics.

The sad truth is that, early in 2016, narcotics were the most commonly prescribed medication in America. I have been appalled to see this develop and refused to participate in the wholesale prescribing of these dangerous medications for benign and chronic pain. **Thousands of Americans are now addicted to prescription narcotics and are dying as a result of overtreatment of benign and chronic pain.**

On February 17, 2016, the AMA president, Dr. Steven J. Stack, wrote, "Over the past 15 years, the nation's opioid epidemic has claimed more than 250,000 lives, according to data from the Centers for Disease Control and Prevention." He has called on physicians to "band together to take specific actions that will turn the tide" (Stack, 2016).

The devastating results from the prescription opiate epidemic include "dependency, addiction, overdose, and death" (Johnson, 2016, p. 31). American narcotic prescriptions have gone from 76 million in 1991 to 219 million in 2011, a 74% increase. The United States has 5% of the world's population but consumes 80% of the world's opiates (Johnson, 2016). Sadly, when a prescribed narcotic is not available to addicted patients, these desperate people may turn to street drugs, including fentanyl and heroin. Besides killing people who have turned to the use of illicit street drugs, narcotic addiction fatalities have also included thousands of accidental prescription overdoses.

It is complicated and time-consuming for a doctor to counsel a patient against the use of narcotics or other addicting drugs. It is difficult to "just say no" to prescribing narcotics as patients plead and beg. It is especially difficult when the patients lack insight into their dependency and perceive the narcotics as safe, while "needing them" to live and function.

Appropriately withholding drugs in the business era of medicine and patient satisfaction surveys leads to angry, hostile, and negative feedback. It is much easier and quicker for a physician to prescribe even a limited number of pills, putting off the definitive, difficult discussion about addiction for another day or another doctor.

While the crisis is only slowly improving, there is hope. The word is being spread far and wide. The prescribing practice of physicians is now being more carefully scrutinized. Physician and patient education alike is providing hope. I am confident that this narcotic abuse epidemic will pass and the tide will recede. As emphasized in the **Preface,** physicians must remember to live by the Hippocratic Oath which includes: "I will apply, for the benefit of the sick, all measures which are required, avoiding those twin traps of overtreatment and therapeutic nihilism."

Engaging in lifelong teaching: I have dedicated my life to practicing medicine while finding the time and energy to teach students and residents. I have also mentored premedical students by having them "shadow" me on rounds and in the clinic.

Although the primary reason I have taught and mentored students is that I felt it was important, I would be disingenuous without admitting that I enjoyed teaching. I love watching the light bulbs go on in students' brains. I love watching students approach a medical diagnostic dilemma for the first time without preconceived notions. I love watching students "connect the dots."

In addition, it is clear to me that the process of staying current and the practice of quality medicine are both enhanced by teaching. Preparing a lecture is more informative for me than attending a speech covering the same material. I have also been blessed over the years with students and medical residents who have rarely shied away from commenting when the teacher "did not practice what he preached." Teaching has, therefore, encouraged me to practice medicine the "right way."

Lifelong Curiosity

A fundamental truth about practicing medicine is that there is invariably more to learn. Realizing this, physicians require lifelong curiosity in order to be successful throughout a medical career. This lifelong thirst for up-to-date medical information and the need to keep abreast of clinically significant advances are essential for physicians, including neurologists.

Continuing lifelong learning: Physicians must be lifelong learners. Medicine is not a fixed body of knowledge that can be learned in training and then used forever.

Because the field of medicine, including the neurosciences, is continually evolving, the successful physician must remain curious throughout his career.

> *"Only the curious will learn and only the resolute overcome the obstacles to learning. The quest quotient has always excited me more than the intelligence quotient."*
>
> *—Eugene S. Wilson*

A practicing clinician researches specific problems for certain individual patients, but cannot routinely investigate the most recent data for every patient every day. A physician is therefore well served to establish a conscientious habit of continuously upgrading his knowledge.

New facts need to be learned, while other learned presumed "truths" proved invalid need to be discarded. Bloodletting is no longer a mainstay treatment option, while other once accepted medical treatments are from time to time discarded. Perhaps it is less well known, for instance, that major, disfiguring breast cancer surgery is no longer known to be efficacious in many patients, because distant metastases occur earlier than once believed.

In neurology, what we know about the brain has doubled approximately every 15 years. Yet, even today, the mysteries of the nervous system seem amazingly daunting, leaving the most brilliant neuroscientists in awe and wonder. I knew practicing neurology would be challenging and it has been. Brain functioning requires an intricate and complex integration of processes to coordinate a vast amount of sensory data, motor commands, cognitive concepts, and emotional states. I was fortunate to be allowed to practice medicine in the neurosciences, which have become even more interesting as the years passed.

I do encourage my students to consider neurology, although they are often intimidated by the complexity of the nervous system. While encouraging students to choose a field of medicine that best fits their unique skill set, I stress that their choice must keep their interest for 40 years. This long view means that their choice does not have to be one that seems easily and quickly mastered.

Many of my colleagues have experienced career burnout. A few years ago, I referred a friend to a capable and accomplished dermatologist. Dermatology is a well-paid specialty, yet has limited disease diversity, no hospital component, and only rarely deals with critical conditions. Clinic visits seldom last more than five to ten minutes. It seems to me that little mystery is hidden from view in a profession dealing with the skin. The consult went well; the advice and treatment were accurate and appropriate. However, my friend noted that my colleague's mood seemed flat and his manner robotic. "Unfortunately," she concluded, "he has been doing his job too long."

My need to get to an answer: While all physicians need to be familiar with the changes in the medical sciences that seem to be coming ever more rapidly, curiosity is especially important. A generalist is taught to focus on what is common and refer patients that might have unusual maladies. The primary care physician typically deals with probabilities, which may dictate a course of treatment without actually confirming a diagnosis.

For example, the vast majority of episodes of lower back pain clear spontaneously. Appropriate primary care encompasses reassurance, a modicum of symptomatic relief, and a follow-up if symptoms persist.

On the other hand, for a patient with lower back pain, a specialist may do a more complete exam, including a careful neurological assessment that may lead to a definitive diagnosis. Taking the extra time to identify the diagnosis is more compatible with my personality makeup. This curiosity is yet another reason that neurology was a good fit for me.

To be clear, a specialist may decide the patient does not have a diagnosis in his field and "sign off the case." A primary care physician continues the care of the patient, no matter the malady diagnosed. A family practitioner in St. Paul, Dr. Kelsey Leonardsmith, epitomizes the primary care physician, the "generalist," who refuses to abandon the patient no matter the diagnosis. When specialists consider a patient only as a diagnostic problem, Kelsey refers to them as "partialists," not a flattering term.

Summary

Learning to successfully practice medicine is more complicated than memorizing facts and passing tests. Besides the acquisition of voluminous amounts of information, a physician must skillfully interpret the patient's history and physical examination findings, perfect the sacrosanct steps to make a diagnosis, and hone the crucial judgment skill set of a clinician. She must learn to formulate a differential diagnosis and treatment plan, while habitually being wary of mistakes and the nuances of the ever-evolving practice of medicine. She must master the effective and efficient use of testing, while clearly understanding the correct interpretation and limitations of the testing results.

The successful practitioner does not just deal with diagnostic puzzles; she also works with people who have problems, pain, and suffering. The successful physician's primary commitment is to her patients, with the goal to improve their lives and eliminate their suffering, while minimizing the negative consequences of treatment regimens like narcotics addiction and unnecessary treatment interventions.

The practice of clinical medicine demands a lifelong curiosity to refine and enrich the physician's knowledge base, while pursuing a journey to keep abreast of medical advancements. For me, it has been easier to remain a lifelong learner while being actively engaged as a lifelong teacher. My students' sense of curiosity and wonder as they attempt to understand the mysteries of the human mind and body has fueled my ongoing enjoyment of medicine while requiring me to always keep my medical knowledge current.

Besides mastering the knowledge and the judgment needed to practice medicine, a clinician also needs to develop the "soft skills" of social-emotional mindfulness, covered in detail in the next chapter.

Chapter 8
Physician Practice Principles: Social-Emotional Mindfulness

It's not a surprise that people-to-people skills are important in the practice of clinical medicine. Consequently, a key to successful physician-patient interaction is a clinician's well-developed social-emotional intelligence. Social-emotional mindfulness is the ability to effectively understand and communicate with people, coupled with the capacity to connect with individual patients and their families. This term encompasses social-emotional awareness and skills.

According to James Runde, author of *Unequaled: Tips for Building a Successful Career Through Emotional Intelligence*, social-emotional intelligence is primarily being mindful of relationships (2016). This naturally starts with a keen sense of self-awareness. Once we have a clear understanding of ourselves, we are better able to self-manage and make responsible decisions. These tools allow the best opportunity to respond effectively to life's challenges and adapt to life's ever-changing conditions.

Physicians also need to focus on having successful relationships with colleagues. Having a keen sense of sincere and respectful collegiality paired with enthusiastic and effective engagement in collaboration with one's associates are key components of mindfulness and the successful practice of medicine (Runde, 2016).

Finally, very importantly, doctors need to establish meaningful relationships with patients. Over the years, I have tried to clarify and continually improve my bedside principles to enable relevant and productive physician-patient communications. These principles include empathy for patients as human beings, enhanced listening skills, a keen sense of rapport building often with use of humor, an advanced ability to counsel and educate patients, and the maintenance of professional honesty.

Some believe that empathy and effective bedside manner are not teachable, although I do not believe that is completely true. Physicians in training are indeed influenced by how they see medicine practiced. Many students, including medical students, are impacted by and try to emulate teachers with advanced communication skills such as the skills discussed in this chapter.

Empathy

The physician who takes time to emotionally connect with patients by understanding their plights often will remain engaged and motivated in the practice of medicine. This emotional connection helps today's physicians cope with a demanding profession undergoing dramatic upheaval, perverse incentives, and fragmented treatment models.

As physicians, we must continue to emotionally connect with our patients, especially those who need our empathy. A patient reminded me, however, to avoid undue "pity party" behavior: "I don't want any sympathy, because in the dictionary the word 'sympathy' is between shit and syphilis."

Listening

> *"The most important thing to do is really listen."*
>
> *—Itzhak Perlman*

Developing the art of listening allows the best chance for the physician-patient interaction to be meaningful. Listening establishes rapport and opens the door to a realistic path forward to fulfilling the physician-patient contract. An advanced listening skill gives the physician a significant head start to understand both the medical and the social issues that typically coexist in a patient encounter.

Listening to patients, family members, and caregivers: After years of reflection, I now believe that listening to patients, their family members, and their caregivers is the key to the successful practice of clinical medicine. It is unfortunate when patients leave a doctor's appointment feeling unheard.

A patient saw six physicians for the feeling of anxiety and a rapid heartbeat. The sixth doctor successfully solved her problem by recommending she stop an over-the-counter weight loss product. When asked why she never mentioned being on this medicine to the other physicians, she said that she had "never been asked." A Joint Commission of Hospital accreditation found that "communication failure (rather than a provider's lack of technical skill) was at the root of over 70% of serious adverse outcomes in hospitals" (Joshi, 2015).

Fulfillment of the physician-patient contract begins with mutual respect and acceptance of responsibility by both the physician and the patient. This starts with respectful listening. To begin the process of taking responsibility for one's health, patients must understand their physician's advice. This understanding starts with accurately hearing what is said. A self-aware man brought his wife to the clinic for a follow-up visit. He introduced her to me by saying, "This is my wife. She is here to hear."

After a career as a medical practitioner, I am absolutely certain that:

- **A physician with excellent listening skills has an advantage in reaching the correct diagnosis.** Careful history taking typically leads to uncovering diagnostic and therapeutic clues that aid the physician's ability to arrive at the correct diagnosis.
- **A physician's ability to listen respectfully can improve the way a patient feels without actually "fixing anything."** A doctor can provide comfort by listening, by "being there" for her patients, and sharing in their grief when apropos. "Being there" for a patient or his family who are overwhelmed by a health crisis allows the physician to add value and comfort, despite lacking the means to affect the outcome of the disease process.
- **A physician's ability to emotionally and intellectually connect with a patient is valuable in and of itself.** People know when their doctor really listens to them and they appreciate it. They feel respected and their concerns validated.
- **A physician provides value when she listens to the family, especially when they are dealing with a loved one with a terminal disease.** Even when the diagnosis and prognosis appear obvious, not all family members may be on the "same page." They may be in different stages of grief and acceptance. Understanding these family dynamics and expectations allows

the physician to provide maximum value to all involved.

- **A physician who listens well typically learns about illnesses in more depth, including the effect on the lives and functioning of their patients.** This knowledge can aid the physician to successfully intervene to improve a patient's life, even when unable to provide a cure.

In my experience, patients who feel listened to are more likely to follow through with the physician's diagnostic and treatment recommendations. These patients are more likely to fulfill their portion of the physician-patient contract.

It is not uncommon for medical students to shun the thought of going into neurology because neurologists "don't fix anything." Indeed, I have "fixed" only a few people in my career. However, significant professional rewards can be reaped when physicians improve people's lives, even without altering the course of their illness. It is the epitome of being human to live productively despite physical and mental disabilities. It is heartwarming to witness individuals thriving despite physical or mental maladies and limitations.

> *"Sometimes it is the artist's task to find out how much music you can still make with what you have left."*
> *—Itzhak Perlman*

Dr. Douglas Wood of the Mayo Clinic put it this way:

> Healthcare does not mean the absence of disease; instead, it means that a person can live life fully and unencumbered. Fundamentally, this means keeping people healthy so that they can meet the needs of those who rely on them, whether their role is that of a father, mother, son, or grandmother (2016, p. 15).

Barriers to listening to patients: Physicians are taught to passively allow patients to tell their stories completely with minimum interruptions. For a myriad of reasons, over time, many physicians become more active in guiding patients through their stories, often formulating differential diagnoses and constructing tentative plans during the patient histories.

As anyone who has been to the doctor recently can verify, the average physician interrupts a patient's history in less than a minute or two. This more active pattern of delineating the history emanates from a belief that the practitioner can add efficiency to a patient's recitation of the story. This may indeed be the case. However, the danger in the physician-guided history is that it can result in an incorrect or incomplete story.

After years in medicine, some practitioners simply lose patience listening to long recitations of a litany of issues, complaints, and worries. Time restraints, the impossibility of trying to follow a patient's narrative, previous experience with a specific patient, quick and often accurate assessments of the situation, or physician arrogance all may contribute to a physician's intolerance to quietly allow a patient to tell the story uninterrupted.

Some patients are indeed poor historians. This is especially common in neurology, where patients are more likely to have brain damage, cognitive impairment, or impaired judgment. At times, behavioral or personality issues can lead to rambling, hard to follow recitations of history. Other patients tell wandering and incoherent stories because they do not know what is important or are confused.

For example, after a man described his ailments to me in detail, his wife sadly admitted, "I would not put a lot of stock in what my husband just told you, doctor. He has a creative recall of past events." Another man describing his neck surgery remarked, "You can't see a surgical scar on the left? Oh, then maybe the surgery was on the right, doc."

Some patients are more worried than ill. One such patient voiced his concern by saying, "I really hope I am sick, because I feel terrible." Another "worried well" individual apologized during his history: "Sorry, I am President of the Ruminators Anonymous Society." Other patients have a lack of medical sophistication or have acquired misinformation that impairs their ability to give a reliable history. After I reassured a patient that she did not have MS, she smiled and admitted her worry emanated from "reading about MS on the internet, convincing me that I had all the symptoms."

An increased emphasis on reaping historical facts from printed or computerized questionnaires is another reason that listening is being discounted in modern medicine. While these questionnaires are constructed to save physician interview time, theoretically aiding a patient to organize his thoughts, it is typically unwise to rely heavily on them. Like myself, many people have difficulty answering questions in a binary fashion without the opportunity to explain the nuances of their situation.

When visiting a hospitalized patient, the doctor must also appear open and anxious to listen. This openness is encouraged when the doctor sits at the bedside. By interviewing the patient while standing, the doctor conveys the rather negative nonverbal message that he is busy and anxious to leave the room.

Fielding unfavorable patient satisfaction scores, one hospital administrator in St. Paul announced a new policy requiring clinicians to sit during all hospital patient visits. When the doctors pointed out that many of the hospital rooms had no chairs for the doctors to use, the embarrassed hospital administrator, who rarely visited patient rooms, vowed to correct this oversight. When the chairs had not arrived a year later, the administrator explained that chairs were expensive due to numerous government-mandated regulations. He sheepishly admitted the hospital had decided to put the new chair expense in a future budget proposal.

Listening to nurses: It's important that a physician be approachable by every medical team member, especially the nurses. Listening to the nurses and their assistants, who spend hours each day with the patients, often reveals useful information and insights.

One day, a nurse quietly handed me the tranquilizers she found in a patient's room that were certainly causing the symptoms that led to admission. I had no idea the patient was on this medication or that she had continued to clandestinely take them while in the hospital.

Many times in my career I have been given credit for a clever diagnosis, when, in fact, the clues were provided by nurses who deserved the credit. Unfortunately, due to a hospital's inherent hierarchy of power, nurses can be reticent to speak up, especially if they question the attending physician.

An intensive care nurse told me about a respirator-dependent patient, whom she felt was regaining consciousness and insight into his situation. An arrogant, disbelieving physician examined the patient roughly and badgered the patient in a demeaning manner. The nurse had to smile when the patient gave the doctor his "middle finger."

Humor

"The physician must have at his command a certain ready wit, as dourness is repulsive both to the healthy and the sick."
—Hippocrates

One might be surprised to see a section about humor in a book written by a neurologist. Neurologists are by reputation rather obsessive-compulsive, studious, detail-oriented, and dry, practicing in a field not distinguished by commonplace or dramatic medical successes. Highlighting that stereotype is the classic neurology joke:

> Two women decided to take a hot air balloon ride. Once up in the air, they quickly realized they were lost. Seeing a man walking on the road below them, they called down to ask where they were. He responded, "You are up in the air in a hot air balloon." One woman turned to the other and remarked, "Our luck to find a neurologist." Shocked by her friend's response, the first woman asked why she thought he was a neurologist. The first woman answered, "He is absolutely precise, accurate, and of no use to us."

Yet, even as a compulsive, fastidious neurologist, I have learned that allowing time for humor is not time wasted. By allowing time for humor (sometimes just wisecracks), I have been able to learn from my patients and about my patients. Using humor and allowing time to listen to my patients to express themselves has, I believe, made me a better physician.

"I like nonsense, it wakes up the brain cells."
—Dr. Seuss

In my practice of neurology, I have been careful to mix humor with the seriousness of dealing with my patients' medical situations. This has highlighted my specific brand of practicing the Art of Medicine. Through humor, I have been able to engage patients in conversation more naturally and spontaneously, often enabling me to genuinely glimpse their level of suffering, gauge their coping mechanisms, and even, at times, come to a more accurate diagnosis. They have, at times, responded in kind. For example, "Have a nice day, Dr. Schanfield, unless you have other plans." Another patient exclaimed, "An apple a day keeps the doctor away, while an onion a day keeps everyone away."

While humor can sometimes be an unhealthy defense mechanism, it can also have a number of positive results. "Studies have shown that humor and laughter lower stress, increase endorphins (thus reducing pain), boost the immune system, and help with coping skills" (Rothschild Levi, 2016). It is widely acknowledged that a positive attitude helps in healing. Patients, families, and the medical staff all respond more positively when the mood is, at least in part, upbeat. On the other hand, angry and despondent patients often seem to do more poorly than expected.

When the medical staff cares for witty, humorous, or optimistic patients, they tend to perform better, although not intentionally, of course. Medical professionals are human and tend to spend more time and energy with patients they enjoy. The extra time can translate into more consistent, conscientious, and complete care. If nurses and doctors dread dealing with a patient, they often discover reasons to shorten their interactions with him.

Because my practice of medicine has emphasized listening, my patients have been allowed to express themselves individually, often in quotable, charming, and humorous ways. Even in the face of serious medical conditions, their concerns with the vicissitudes of illness and death have been laced with funny observations and witty insights. As a physician caring for thousands of patients over the course of 40 years, I recall many humorous moments, as these precious vignettes have increased the richness of my life as a practicing neurologist. This should not be discounted, as it has helped insulate me from professional burnout.

> *"If I were given the opportunity to present a gift to the next generation, it would be the ability for each individual to learn to laugh at himself."*
> *—Charles Schultz*

Relaxed Compulsiveness

I have enjoyed my patients and allowed my joy to be obvious. Physician-patient encounters can be stressful. Striving to relax a nervous, worried, or anxious patient is generally worth the effort. I label the ambiance encompassing my practice of medicine as "relaxed compulsiveness." This seemingly paradoxical and amusingly ironic phrase often puzzles the medical residents and students.

My goal has been to practice medicine with a seemingly natural, unhurried, and pleasant demeanor, engaging my patients, rather than lecturing them. I have chosen to use humor and charm whenever possible. One definition of success could be a 90-year-old patient bringing dark chocolate candy to each office visit because I reminded her of "my sweet, deceased husband."

I have encouraged each patient to smile or laugh, attempting to make them comfortable and relaxed as they tell their stories, with as little tension and nervousness as possible. To convey a sense of relaxed joy successfully, I have had to avoid appearing dismissive, lackadaisical, and unconcerned.

Working to relax a patient and the family should not be interpreted as disrespecting the patient, minimizing the seriousness of the medical concerns, or suggesting a less than assiduous evaluation and treatment approach to the problem. Lightening the mood during a patient interview should not be interpreted as permission to the students and medical residents to be less industrious in addressing each patient's concerns and issues.

Medical residents and students have sometimes misinterpreted my relaxed bedside manner as a sign of nonchalance in my approach to diagnosis and treatment. I have been clear that establishing a relaxed ambiance does not relieve our medical team of the responsibility to be conscientiously thorough. No matter the situation, I have endeavored to gain rapport with each patient, while meticulously analyzing every issue step by step.

Bringing humor to the bedside also may lead to a small modicum of immediate happiness. One of my good friends, Dr. Michael Neren, likes to remind me that a physician's primary role is to improve a patient's life. Bringing a smile to a patient enhances that person's life transiently, and may even alter their long-term outcome.

Counseling, Educating, and Advising

It is important to emphasize that physicians do more than diagnose, consult surgeons, or recommend medical treatments. This is especially important for neurologists, who typically deal with numerous diseases that are chronic and progressive, some with known causes and treatments but many without.

A mindful physician continually enhances her facility for counseling, informing, educating, advising, and providing support. To effectively provide meaningful communication and emotional support, the physician cannot rely on the use of a "one size fits all" formula or a cookbook approach to medicine. Most patients and families benefit from individualized approaches and methods.

We should expect a physician to provide effective advice and counsel if she:

- Has a good working knowledge of the personality of the patient and the family.
- Has significant insight into where the patient and family are along the continuum of acceptance of, for example, the diagnosis of a fatal brain tumor, Parkinson's Disease, Alzheimer's Disease, or Multiple Sclerosis.
- Is allowed sufficient time by our medical system for such human and humane interactions.
- Intimately understands how the illness directly and indirectly affects a particular patient and family.

Dr. Barbara K. Lipska, a neuroscientist who unfortunately developed malignant melanoma brain metastases, highlighted this final point. After treatment, the scientist's confusion cleared, leading her to realize that "I felt I understood for the first time what many of the patients I study go through—the fear and confusion of living in a world that doesn't make sense; a world in which the past is forgotten and the future is utterly unpredictable" (2016).

Professional Honesty

Another tenet of Dr. Neren's view of quality medical care is that patients are entitled "to good care provided respectfully and appropriately with consent, while receiving sufficient information to understand that they have received good medical care" (personal communication, April 2016). Of course, he is correct.

Physicians must strive to guarantee that patients and their families are well informed as to the diagnosis and treatment options. Physicians must strive to guarantee that each patient has given his informed consent.[32] To do this successfully, physicians must excel at the art of medicine while using their social-emotional

[32] Informed consent, a fundamental principle of healthcare, refers to the process whereby the patient and the clinician engage in a dialogue about a proposed medical treatment's nature, consequences, harms, benefits, risks, and alternatives.

intelligence. To do this well, physicians must convey the meaningful information at the right time with clarity laced with empathy.

Over time, however, doctors may become jaded, treating people as illnesses instead of individuals with illnesses, as repeatedly emphasized in this book. It is not uncommon for a physician to begin to "protect" herself from emotionally identifying with patients. It can be emotionally disabling for a clinician to watch random illnesses destroy people's lives and those of their families. It goes without saying that considerably less personal risk exists for the doctor who remains aloof, creating a professional barrier between the clinician and the patients, who are suffering in the throes of physical and/or emotional crises.

Besides potentially eroding a physician's personal sense of well-being, allowing a significant emotional connection with patients could theoretically interfere with a doctor's ability to maintain intellectual objectivity. However, I believe that intellectual objectivity can be maintained without sacrificing compassion and empathy. After laughing and crying with me about her fatal disease, a woman confessed, "Thanks, doc. I now realize that I am not going through this alone and I am actually doing better than I deserve."

After learning to identify my emotions, I have avoided erecting insulating barriers between my patients and me. I have learned that I could cry at times with families and allow myself to feel pain and grief triggered by their losses, illnesses, and deaths. I believe that continuing to care has kept my practice of medicine meaningful, real, and alive. Patients know when their doctor cares. Patients know when their doctor is intellectually and emotionally invested in their well-being.

A colleague recently reminded me of a shared hospitalized patient who had suffered a devastating stroke. The distraught wife pleaded with us to say that her husband was going to be fine. I sadly and silently looked at her and gave her a hug. She burst into tears, hugged me back, and thanked us for being honest while providing the best treatment available.

Yet, physicians need to balance being empathetic and caring without "bringing it home." Despite laughing and crying with patients and their families, I have been able to keep my personal life separate from my professional life. To experience empathy safely, a physician who allows human connections to trigger appropriate emotional responses must be mindful and self-aware. He must be mindful of his emotional responses to patient crises, allowing him to realistically separate his family life from that of the patients.

In other words, being self-aware aids the clinician to identify his emotions and prevent them from interfering with his personal life. Prolonged grieving with patients, especially when unrecognized, will dampen a doctor's joy in living and practicing medicine, risking professional burnout and mood disorders.

Having conversations about bad news: Sharing bad news with patients and their families is challenging and emotional. "The physician's duty," according to Dr. Paul Kalanithi, "is not to always stave off death or return patients to their old lives, but to take into our arms a patient and family whose lives have disintegrated and work until they can stand back up and face what makes sense of their own existence" (2016, p. 166).

Physicians often avoid this crucial, difficult task in different ways. Dr. Kathleen Kieran from the University of Washington and Seattle Children's Hospital suggests "both patients and clinicians may create an environment where breaking bad news is avoided." She laments what she calls the "MUM effect" that "reflects a dislike of giving bad news" (2016, p. 29).

Alternatively, Dr. Kieran discourages "dumping." This occurs when a physician dumps bad news on the patient and family by reciting the facts and then immediately departing. This occurred to one of my patients during a first meeting with a neuro-oncologist who said, "For your brain tumor, the treatments include radiation and chemotherapy. I doubt either will work, but we will begin them tomorrow." The neuro-oncologist then walked out of the consultation room, presumably oblivious to the trauma he had caused and not knowing that the patient's family fired him.

I have long pondered why some specialists, such as the oncologist above, with little explanation repeatedly recommend to dying patients new treatments with minimal rewards, high likelihood of complications, and unjustified expense. Every potentially terminally ill patient is entitled to an honest discussion of the positives and negatives of new proposed treatments, especially when the known and established effective treatments have failed.

Such in-depth conversations are certainly discouraged by our system of financial incentives, which provides little remuneration for prolonged counseling sessions. The system rewards "doing something," like surgery, chemotherapy, or radiation therapy.

It often takes less physician time to recommend a new medical trial that is unlikely to succeed rather than to honestly admit that all hope is lost, hospice is the only reasonable next step, and death is imminent.

If a new, life-changing diagnosis exists, I believe that a physician has an obligation to say so, being careful to choose the appropriate time. The timing and content of conveying such a devastating prognosis depends upon each patient and family. Individual patients have a wide variation in their psychological makeup and their ability to absorb bad news. People are ready for the truth at different times. Being honest does not demand the physician be dogmatically hopeless while conveying bad news.

In my experience, patients often have more capacity for understanding dire circumstances than physicians or their families recognize. One of my patients in such a terminal state smiled and said, "Now that I am in hospice, the staff and nurses are wonderful. I get massages whenever I wish, lots of God-shrink talk, and all the drugs I want for free."

After going on palliative care, another delightful man in the office introduced me to his family by saying, "Here is my family, who I now refer to as 'my dope ring.'" I have found it comforts patients and their families when I follow a declaration of a sad or hopeless prognosis with a small modicum of optimism by saying, "I do honestly hope that you will, in the future, tell me that I was overly pessimistic with today's dire prediction."

> ***"A tureen of tragedy was best allotted by the spoonful as few patients demand the whole at once. Most need time to digest."***
> ***—Paul Kalanithi***

Dr. Kieran believes that few physicians are formally trained to give bad news humanely, successfully, and at the right time. Physicians must be trained to meet people where they are and when they are ready. She has published a six-step **SPOKES method** to humanely convey devastating news:

1. **S**et up the interview.
2. Assess the patient's **P**erception.
3. **O**btain the patient's invitation to proceed further with the discussion.
4. Impart **K**nowledge and information to the patient.

5. Address the patient's **E**motions with **E**mpathic responses.
6. Conclude by **S**ummarizing the **S**trategy. (Kieran, 2016, p. 28)

An acquaintance died of cancer at a very young age. At his last oncology visit, his doctor made it clear that all treatment protocols had failed, quietly announced that "there is nothing left to be done," and walked out of the examining room. The man and his family, who were obviously saddened by the news, were shocked by the abruptness of this pronouncement.

After thoughtful reflection, this man accepted his fate, yet took action by going home to make a list of "what was yet to be done." This was a list written by a human being dying of cancer, not a medical practitioner. His list included people he wanted to see and spend time with, conversations he wished to have, an ethical will he was determined to write, affairs that needed to be put in order, and how he planned to fill each remaining day. He left a road map on how to live and how to die with dignity for his friends, family, and especially his children. It turned out that there was "a lot left to do."

End-of-life talks with patients are rarely easy. Some patients and families may never accept the truth, while others need time. Hopefully, after periods of denial, anger, bargaining, and depression, most work their way to acceptance.[33]

Typically in complex, incurable medical conditions, patients receive a lot of advice from friends and family, whether requested or not. Some advice is good and some is not. Some of the information can be helpful, with some filled with inaccuracies and false hope. Unfortunately, patients may even stumble across fraudulent medical providers seeking only to profit from their misfortune.

A patient of mine clearly understood what we had discussed, including the diagnosis and the prognosis. She later told me with a sad smile, "I received a second opinion from my daughter that was much more upbeat than yours, doctor. It was free and very likely worth every penny."

A 25-year-old woman suffered a massive stroke. To save her life, I recommended a neurosurgeon remove half of the young woman's skull to make room for the

[33] Denial, anger, bargaining, depression, and acceptance are the five stages of grief, as identified by Elisabeth Kübler-Ross in *On Death and Dying* (1969).

inevitable brain swelling, which, if untreated, would be fatal. During this crisis, I honestly confided with the young woman's parents that I feared, even with the surgery, her recovery could be very limited. Yet, not every dire prediction turns out to be accurate, especially in the young. As is my tradition, I followed my dire warning with an honest hope that I was being overly pessimistic. We all agreed to continue aggressive care, including any and all interventions possible to keep this young woman alive.

Despite this young woman's prolonged hospital stay with a myriad of medical issues, including ten days of coma, she and her mother walked into my office for a follow-up appointment three months later. Although she needed a cane, suffered left arm and leg weakness, and could not see to the left, she was smiling, thinking clearly, and happy to be alive. She, her parents, and I were all thrilled that my warning that she might not have a meaningful recovery proved to be overly pessimistic. When I last saw her, she continued to enjoy life despite her obvious disability and was trying to find her place in life.

Physicians sometimes disappear from a case when all is lost, because "there is nothing left to do." In my experience, there is often much a physician can and should do. A physician with nothing left "to fix" can be needed at the bedside of a dying patient, providing value by answering questions, conveying useful information, and lending support. One such role is to counsel families on how to say goodbye to their dying loved one by following these five steps:

1. "We love you."
2. "You have lived a worthwhile life that is appreciated."
3. "We will be okay without you."
4. "We will miss you."
5. "If I have made you angry or upset, I apologize." Alternatively, "I forgive you for . . ."

Discussing bad news and/or end of life with patients and families is rarely easy. Some patients and families may never accept the truth, while others need time to do so. After periods of denial, anger, bargaining, and depression, most will hopefully work their way to acceptance with the help of their physician.

Facing uncertainty and mistakes: I have previously highlighted the importance of a physician's periodic re-evaluation of a chosen diagnosis or treatment plan to avoid encountering dead ends or misguided treatment paths. This takes courage, adaptability, humility, and self-awareness, all tenets of social-emotional intelligence.

While the process of re-examining prior judgments is important, honestly facing actual medical mistakes is essential. These practices contribute to improved medical care, while hopefully not degrading the physician's long-term decision-making skills by injuring his ego. It can indeed be tricky to appropriately question previous decisions and admit mistakes, yet remain a confident physician.

Sound clinical judgment is one of the bedrocks of a successful medical practice, which must incorporate a physician's realistic self-awareness of his skill set and its limitations, while maintaining an appropriate amount of self-confidence and ego. Both overconfidence and lack of confidence are incompatible with the practice of high-quality medicine.

A diagnostician typically flirts with error when he skips steps. Certainly, physicians should strive to efficiently practice medicine, and a rigid approach to diagnosis is not usually necessary. However, jumping to conclusions because of time restraints, overconfidence, fatigue, or laziness is fraught with danger. When taking a diagnostic shortcut, the professional must be certain that he has enough personal information to account for the patient's individual uniqueness.

> *"The decision is often difficult, the occasion fleeting and the experience liable to error."*
>
> *—Hippocrates*

While it is rarely emphasized, an outstanding diagnostician must learn from his mistakes. Once a medical mistake has been made, the clinician's first step is to admit that a mistake has occurred. To admit a mistake happened sounds rather mundane, but it can be difficult. Physicians are obviously not paid to make mistakes.

In addition, threat of malpractice is real and may influence a practitioner's willingness to admit errors, whether or not he was actually at fault. Many mistakes do not lead to harm. If harm has occurred, however, the stakes are clearly higher. Even without malpractice, a doctor's reputation may suffer if the situation is not handled with care. Good reputations take years to establish, but may be lost in an instant.

Fortunately, it has been my experience that patients tend to forgive physician mistakes if openly acknowledged with a sincere apology. Forgiveness is especially forthcoming if the patient has felt listened to, felt respected, and believes the physician has been conscientious and caring. Patients appreciate a physician who is honest, respectful, empathetic, and humble.

After admitting that a mistake has occurred, the second step is for the physician to gain insight into how things could have been managed differently and convey this information to the patient and family. Patients and their families appreciate reassurances that knowledge has been gained from the medical error, which will be used to avoid similar events in the future.

For example, I may have been misled by an incorrect radiologist interpretation. It would be easy in this circumstance to blame the radiologist, while learning nothing from the case. Looking to learn from the situation, my take-away lesson has typically been that I put "too much stock" in the radiologist's reading.

Another example is of a patient who did not reveal a crucial historical fact, such as a medication allergy that triggered a medical crisis. Again, it would be easy to blame the patient and learn nothing from the case. In this scenario, my take-away lesson has been that my process of extracting the patient history should be improved.

> ***"I have clearly recorded this: for one can learn good lessons also from what has been tried but clearly has not succeeded, when it is clear why it has not succeeded."***
> ***—Hippocrates***

Penny Hodges-Goetz, an experienced neurosurgery nurse practitioner, wisely questions her peers, "Do you want to appear right or do you want to get it right now and in the future?" A professional should strive to gain new knowledge and insight from each case, whether handled appropriately or not.

It is easy to accept praise when things go well. It is easy to accept compliments when the outcome is good. It is easy to accept credit for reaching a correct diagnosis or formulating a creative and effective treatment strategy. However, it is hard to admit mistakes. Unfortunately, some physicians find it harder to admit mistakes the longer they practice medicine. This need not be the case. The ego of the established physician needs to be formidable enough to admit mistakes, while striving to learn from each error in judgment, missed diagnosis, or mistake.

A Migraine In Room 3, A Stroke In Room 4

It is widely acknowledged that medical errors are typically 85% a process problem and 15% a people problem, which should make it rather painless to learn from medical failures, as well as successes. Unfortunately, this remains a significant problem.

According to the Institute of Medicine report of September 2015, diagnostic errors in medicine are like a "blind spot in healthcare." These errors lead to 10% of all deaths and 6% to17% of hospital adverse events. The Physician Insurers Association of America (PIAA) lists diagnostic errors as a prevalent factor in about a third of neurology lawsuits (Fallik, 2016b, p. 8).

It takes a significant amount of social-emotional mindfulness for a physician to allow patients to see his uncertainty while maintaining self-confidence. Each physician should honestly differentiate situations in which they know, in which they think they know, and in which they are uncertain. To openly balance honesty and self-confidence is tricky for an experienced physician; it is even more difficult to teach to students and medical residents.

After completing my training program, I entered the private practice of neurology in St. Paul. During my first year, a man came to me for what he announced was a work-related injury manifested by right arm and shoulder pain. Although his job was physically demanding, no clear work injury could be diagnosed. He was previously healthy, although he was a middle-aged smoker, which increased his risk for lung disease, including cancer. Lung cancer, which turned out to be the cause of his symptoms, can present with arm and shoulder pain if the cancer has spread to involve the nerves under the shoulder. Unfortunately, I did not make the correct diagnosis.

In retrospect, I was misled by his insistence that his symptoms were work-related and his X-ray was normal. The outside records later revealed that the X-ray was indeed normal, but it was of his right shoulder and not of his chest. By the time I had clarified the X-ray issue, he had coughed up blood, leading his primary doctor to correctly diagnose cancer. I missed the diagnosis of the lung cancer, which had indeed grown into the nerves under his shoulder.

The patient and I discussed his case in follow-up. I apologized and promised to review outside X-rays in a more timely fashion in the future. I felt terrible, although he forgave me. I took little solace from the literature revealing that lung cancer is incurable once it has invaded the nerve bundle under the shoulder.

I also recall misdiagnosing a patient as having ALS (Amyotrophic Lateral Sclerosis or Lou Gehrig's Disease), which is fatal. Fortunately, I referred him to the University of Minnesota Department of Neurology for a second opinion where a neurology subspecialty colleague determined that the man had a treatable condition and recommended treatment. I owned my mistake and apologized to the patient and his wife, who was a nurse. Following this difficult conversation, the patient chose to continue his treatment at our offices for the next ten years, until I retired. We have been so very pleased that the treatment has dramatically normalized his functioning.

To make a mistake is human and I have made mistakes. My connection with my patients has sustained me when I have made mistakes. My patients have recognized that I have done my best and have forgiven me. This human connection, which comes directly from having patients feel they have been listened to, respected, and valued, has also sustained me when accused unjustifiably of harming or mistreating a patient.

I was unjustifiably sued for medical malpractice 30 years ago. Yet, even when it is clear that a lawsuit is without merit, physicians fret and lose sleep when they are sued. I was no exception. The lawsuit was based on the delay in diagnosing and treating a herniated lumbar disc. At the time, MRI imaging of the lumbar spine was in its infancy. The official radiology report incorrectly diagnosed a nerve root tumor. The actual diagnosis was an unusual, laterally located herniated disc.[34]

The patient's back pain radiated down her leg in a fashion rather typical for a herniated disc, causing her to be miserable. I referred the patient to a St. Paul neurosurgeon. Despite the patient being miserable and the husband requesting immediate surgery, the surgeon hesitated to operate, fearing the possibility of a tumor, and instead ordered another test, a CT-Myelogram[35]. The patient and her husband wanted immediate relief, sought a second opinion, and were able to convince a university neurosurgeon to operate immediately. A herniated disc was found, rather than a tumor, with the surgery immediately relieving the pain.

During the follow-up in my office, the patient seemed pleased with her outcome as she had no pain and her examination was normal. After my explanation, the patient expressed no hostility. Unbeknownst to me, her husband, who did not come to the

[34] The herniated disc fragment slipped so far laterally that it appeared completely separate from the main body of the disc itself, leading the radiologist to suggest incorrectly that it was a tumor.

[35] A CT-Myelogram is an alternative way of imaging the spine by injecting a dye in the spinal canal, then doing CT imaging of the area.

follow-up office visit, remained angry that we had allowed his wife to suffer an extra two weeks until he had arranged for a successful surgery. When the operating neurosurgeon would not testify against me, the lawsuit was dismissed without a trial.

Fortunately, since those early days, MRI scans have dramatically improved, making this type of confusion unlikely.

Summary

The successful practice of medicine is predicated upon incorporating an enormous body of knowledge and a significant complement of social-emotional intelligence. While rarely taught, social-emotional mindfulness is critical to the clinical practice of medicine.

To be an accomplished clinician, a physician must experience empathy for his patients, and master the art of listening, counseling, and advising patients and their families. She must remain honest and humble, admit uncertainty, accept blame when appropriate, and apologize when pertinent.

She should resist the temptation to shun emotional connections with patients in the name of self-preservation and not shy away from conveying bad news in a respectful, humane way at the right time.

Personally, I have found it remarkably useful to employ an upbeat mood when possible, sprinkled with therapeutic "doses" of humor. I have found it essential to remain compulsively thorough and conscientious, and to treat each individual with respect. Stated in another way, the job is serious, yet the physician should not take himself too seriously.

It cannot be over emphasized how difficult, yet how crucial, it is for a physician to have an appropriate degree of confidence as well as humility and the strength of character to honestly admit mistakes and learn from them. Following these guiding principles and developing the social-emotional skill set they are founded upon, a physician will experience a true sense of joy, fulfillment, and satisfaction, while mitigating the chance of succumbing to professional burnout.

Part 3

LIFE LESSONS FROM MY PATIENTS

Since early in my career, I placed a premium on listening to patients express themselves as individuals. This has enhanced my professional life, while minimizing career burnout. It became clear that the patients were educating me. They were teaching me valuable lessons about life, while serving as role models as they wrestled with illness, aging, and death. Understanding what my patients were providing me led me to collect patient quotes and stories, which served as the basis of this book.

In **Chapter 9,** I recall many of my patients' descriptions of living with illness and aging that were remarkably laced with humor, charm, and wit. They in turn encouraged me not to forsake the benefits of humor.

In addition, I loved recording my patients' observations concerning life, family, work, and relationships, spelled out in **Chapter 10.** It also seemed reasonable to review in **Chapter 10** my approach to and joy of having children and teenagers as patients in the office.

Chapter 11 begins with a review of the challenges in diagnosing and treating the elderly, followed by memories of my senior patients, some patients thriving and some patients failing. It has been my privilege to document glimpses of their journey as they faced aging and death with courage, persistence, humor, and acceptance. **Chapter 11** did not feel complete without two sections on dying young: one with warning and one without warning.

Chapter 9
Patients' Humor

"Among those whom I like or admire, I can find no common denominator, but among those whom I love, I can: all of them make me laugh."

—W. H. Auden

Because my practice of medicine has emphasized listening, my patients have been allowed to express themselves individually, often in quotable, endearing, and humorous ways. Even in the face of serious medical conditions, their concerns with the vicissitudes of illness and death have, at times, been laced with funny observations and witty insights. How memorable to recall a patient retell this hospital admission story: "Who should we contact in case of an emergency, sir?" asked the hospital admissions clerk. My patient honestly responded, "Anyone in hearing range would be great."

It has been my privilege to care for many brave and likeable people, who have faced disease and disability without losing their humanity and refusing to become marginalized.

Multiple Sclerosis: I have treated hundreds of patients with MS, a disease characterized by attacks of weakness, clumsiness, numbness, bladder control issues, and/or visual loss. Early in the disease, these attacks often clear. However, over time, physical limitations begin to accumulate, leading to various amounts of disability. Currently, no cure exists, although we now have excellent drugs that dramatically decrease the attacks and slow the progression of disability. Imagine the chutzpah[36] it takes to joke about one's own health induced-limitations when suffering from a condition like MS. For example:

- A woman with MS developed an essentially useless left arm. She quipped, "I keep my arm around only for looks."
- A middle-aged woman with gait difficulties acknowledged with an ironic smile, "My high heel days are now exceedingly limited."
- A man suggested that his gait difficulties had advanced so far that "my middle name should be Fall."
- A 40-year-old MS patient with a clumsy, wobbly walk thought about making a bumper sticker that reads: "Hire the handicapped. You will have fun watching them walk."
- An impotent man with MS explained, "It's like being able to get to the fire, but then being unable to get the water hose up to the fire."
- "Walking on my bilaterally spastic legs," said another patient, "probably looks like an old-fashioned egg beater."
- A patient with advanced MS suffered intermittent trouble initiating voiding, yet, at other times, would wet herself "out of the blue." She decided that she was "suffering from keep-age and leakage."
- MS patients often suffer from a dramatic fatigue, as if someone physically drained their bodies of energy. One patient described this fatigue this way: "I get so weak that my husband pours me onto the couch and the TV watches me rest."
- After suffering a particularly vicious flare-up of her MS, a woman remained weak and wobbly exclaimed, "I have become a snapdragon. I have snapped and now I'm dragging."

Parkinson's Disease: Another common neurological disease is Parkinson's Disease, initially described as the "Shaking Palsy" in 1817 by Sir James A. Parkinson. Remarkably, my patients, at times, have faced this progressive, degenerative condition with realistic, endearing insights:

- "Now that I have Parkinson's Disease, I feel like I'm trapped in a lazy body."

---

[36] Chutzpah is Yiddish for supreme self-confidence.

- "Because of my gait difficulty from Parkinson's Disease, my cane is a brake, so I don't keep going faster and faster forward till I fall."
- "I am a level-headed Swede that does not take sides. I drool out of both sides of my mouth equally."
- "I can go awhile, but then I must rest awhile."

Not every patient with a tremor has Parkinson's Disease. One patient was referred to me for Parkinson's Disease, but instead had the more benign syndrome of Familial Tremor. He commented, "My tremor runs in the family. We use it as a weed whacker."

Degenerative Arthritis: Many physicians help people cope with degenerative arthritis, which is a widespread condition that becomes increasingly common, even crippling, as we age. Some people are able to cope with the pain and disability better than others:

- "I pay my bills sitting down," said a severely arthritic 80-year-old man, "because I feel like a million bucks sitting and not worth a damn nickel standing up."
- Another man remarked, "My back is bad enough that I'm thinking about renting it out."
- A woman suffering from the steadily worsening arthritic changes of aging said, "My arthritic knuckles are monuments to my long-standing, painful arthritis."
- One man, who suffered through physical therapy for his stiff and painful legs, declared, "I realize that it is no coincidence that 'therapy' and 'torture' both start with 'T' and both have seven letters."

To determine if the degenerative disc disease causes damage to the nerves and muscles, it is not uncommon for a neurologist to perform a test called an electromyography (EMG). An EMG involves shocks and needles, and is not without discomfort. After one of my patients finished the exam, he grumbled and laughed, "It's a good thing your office has a sign out front announcing that the clinic bans guns, doctor!"

As one patient bluntly summed it up, "Life is funny, but mostly not."

Gait Difficulties: Throughout this book, I have stressed that patients are people with illness, not examples of disease. To listen to patients explain how progressive medical conditions disrupt their normal daily living is to receive an education not provided in the medical textbooks. For instance, my neurology patients have described their gait difficulties in many unique ways:

- "I now attempt to have a controlled stumble."
- "I have fallen so many times that my son says that I'm making an art form out of falling."
- "I tripped and fell on a busy sidewalk, as I tend to do a lot these days," said an 89-year-old woman. "This time, an elderly man tried to stop my fall, but was unsuccessful and fell on top of me. I guess men are still falling for me."
- "Yes, I need a power chair to get around, but don't call it an electric chair, because that is reserved for convicted criminals."
- "Fortunately, I prefer my marbles over mobility."
- "I now walk or move like a snail."

Dementia: Remarkably, even some patients suffering from dementia, most commonly caused by Alzheimer's Disease, have joked with me:

- "I'm not bad off, as I only have 'half-zheimer's' disease."
- "As a neurologist, you have a big task just to find my brain."
- "I know I did not very accurately draw that three-dimensional square you asked me to draw as part of the memory test, doctor. Despite not being able to do that, please remember I made a pretty darn good living for years, enabling us to raise four children and send them all to college."
- "I realize I recalled only three of four things you asked me to memorize, but you should be happy with that, doc. I am."
- "I'm not confused really, as I believe my brain works fine. I just can't find the set of directions."
- "It feels like my brain is like new . . . never been used."
- Dementia patients seem to have a variable amount of insight into their advancing cognitive decline. One brilliant, yet forgetful man, with some insight, smirked as he said, "I don't think, thereafter I am not."
- "I can't think of anything I have forgotten lately."

One of my dear friends unfortunately became my patient. A brilliant teacher and school counselor, she was fastidious in her use of language. She died of autopsy-proven Alzheimer's Disease. It is now known that well-educated patients can cope with cognitive decline for years with less apparent disability, as was the case for my friend. In an attempt to rule out other conditions, she underwent a brain MRI about two years before her death. The MRI was technically difficult to perform as her prominent kyphoscoliosis[37] prevented positioning her optimally in the scanner due to her inability to lie flat. The MRI technician, therefore, asked, "Please lay on your left side." Despite having advanced Alzheimer's Disease, she somewhat haughtily responded, "No. My dear young man, chickens lay eggs; people lie on one side or the other."

Stroke: I have learned that patients' abilities to cope and accept the difficulties that life presents are highly variable. For a new stroke patient, best medical practice recommends withholding food until a speech pathologist guarantees that the risk of aspiration and subsequent pneumonia is low. Hospitals are not typically staffed 24-7 with qualified speech therapists, so some patients may wait a day or more to be cleared to eat. Upon experiencing such a delay, one patient smiled, winked, and declared, "I was so hungry last night, I dreamed that I ate a five-pound marshmallow and awoke to find my pillow missing."

Another stroke patient required additional heart tests. After hearing the complicated results of her tests, she smirked and summarized, "I guess my heart monitoring was normal with some abnormalities."

Headaches: Neurologists commonly evaluate patients with headaches, including migraines and tension headaches. Many patients can cope, while others have difficulties; some respond to medications and some do not; some understand the cause of the headaches and some do not:

- "My migraine lifetime motto: Pain in the head, go to bed."
- "My chronic headaches have been helped by that new medicine. It's unbelievable the amount of headaches I don't have any longer."
- Trying to get to the root of a man's rather prominent tension headache syndrome, I questioned him about stress. He responded, "Doc, let me answer your question this way. Do I have stress? My best man ran off with my fiancé. Do I smoke? Yes. Do I drink alcohol? Absolutely!"

---

[37] Kyphoscoliosis is an abnormal curvature of the spine, combining scoliosis (her spine was "S"-shaped) with an excessive convex curvature of the spine (a forward flexion at the waist).

- A woman was brought to me for her headaches, but seemed unconcerned: "I don't appear worried, doctor, because I am paying you to worry about me."

Miscellaneous conditions: The grace and charm with which some of my patients have accepted medical conditions, whether minor, serious, or life-changing, has been memorable, sometimes inspirational, and occasionally hilarious. I have applauded my patients when they embrace life with gusto despite the limitations of serious illness. It certainly is healthier to laugh than to wallow in self-pity and sadness. Many of my patients have reminded me of this:

- "My toes were amputated so that I could be closer to the free throw line."
- "My open-heart surgery has improved my cleavage," said a 75-year-old woman.
- "I have PISS: pregnancy induced stupidity syndrome."
- "There is so much tingling in my body that it sounds like I'm playing *Jingle Bells*."
- "I have to laugh when my dizzy spells occur, as it feels like my head is a bowling ball on a bendy, thin straw."
- "My hot flashes are so bad that my glasses fog up," said one woman, who referred to herself as "a red hot mama."
- A balding man, who only had hair on the sides of his head, joked, "I grew too tall to keep the top of my head covered with hair."
- One unusual man announced that he was a longtime sufferer of optical rectitis. When I suggested there was no such disease, he clarified it for me: "The nerve to my eye is connected to my rectum, doc, giving me a shitty outlook on life."

Of course, even as we age, many episodes of illnesses are reversible and benign. One such process is called Transient Global Amnesia, an unusual disorder highlighted by a sudden, but temporary period (usually lasting hours) of complete loss of short-term memory, while all other cognitive abilities remain intact. The amnesia clears completely without permanent brain damage spontaneously without treatment. After one such bout, a patient's wife smiled, shook her head, and remarked, "My husband has totally recovered from his bout of amnesia as you promised, doctor, but he still has no common sense."

Aging into the Golden Years: The concept of the "golden years" promises relief from stress, an enjoyable retirement, and peaceful days spent reminiscing on the porch with friends and family, fishing, and communing with nature at the cabin. Joking about his advancing age, instead of saying he was 88 years of age, a patient said, "My age is 39 x 2 + 10." In a similar vein, another elderly man responded to the question of how old he was by saying, "November 3rd is the 42nd anniversary of my 39th birthday."

During the golden years, fortunate seniors have less worry about money and love. With good fortune, many have unhurried time to spend with friends, family, and especially grandchildren. However, as we age, medical conditions become more common, progressive, and unfixable. Advanced age is not a disease, but medical maladies become more common with age. My patients have frequently reminded me of the realities of aging, sometimes with realism couched in charm and wit:

- "These are not the golden years; everything hurts and nothing works."
- "I'd prefer vanilla if these are indeed the golden years."
- Cherishing one aspect of death, one man announced, "My gravestone will say, 'No more lists.'"
- "My personal trainer might know stuff and heaven knows I need help, but really I have underwear older than her."

Of course, not every elderly patient does poorly in their golden years. One patient remarked, "If I felt any better, I would probably have to take something for it."

Unintended humor: Some of my humorous patient vignettes were unintentionally funny. With dementia, confusion tends to occur more frequently at night when it is dark. This disorientation and confusion is often referred to as "sundowning." One of my patients made me smile by mistakenly referring to this as "Sunday-downing." Other examples include:

- After we agreed that a woman's 88-year-old husband should be placed in a nursing home, she asked, "Who will help me open tight jelly jars?" Her calm and unflappable husband replied, "Jammed if I know."
- As a person's cognitive abilities fail, thought becomes more concrete and less nuanced. For example, when asked how he slept, a man responded seriously and objectively, "On my back."
- A 78-year-old woman was becoming forgetful, yet kept trying to live nor-

mally. Her daughter was disturbed to learn that her mother had been recently stopped for speeding. When the policeman asked to see her license, she responded a bit haughtily, "Please, officer, I wish you guys would make up your mind. Last week, one of your partners took it away from me."

- A fastidious, elderly woman remarked, "I am not sure that it was a good idea to have this cataract surgery. Now I see all this dirt and dust in the house that I did not know was there."
- A nursing home resident suffered some memory loss with significant mood fluctuations. His daughter faithfully visited him late each afternoon after work. Despite the nurses saying he typically awakened refreshed, cheerful, and pleasant, he would often yell at her. When his daughter asked why he would selectively and regularly yell at her, he responded, "I suppose that by the time you get here each day, someone has pissed me off."
- A man's wife set up his pill case each week to encourage his medication compliance. I was dumbfounded when he admitted to me privately that, at week's end, he would secretly replace the forgotten pills back in the original pill bottles so his wife would not worry.
- A good friend, Karyl, arranged to take her father and his memory-impaired nursing home roommate to Thanksgiving dinner. When she arrived, the two men were not ready, so it took a while for her to help them finish getting dressed. When they were finally ready to go, the roommate said, "Karyl, thank you for a most wonderful and delicious Thanksgiving dinner." To which Karyl replied, "George, we have not yet left for dinner."

Summary

The practice of medicine is about people and that is as it should be. It is my opinion that when our system allows time for intimate physician-patient interactions, both the patients and the physicians are advantaged. The patients benefit when they feel respected as individuals, especially when encouraged to tell their story in their own words. Although sadness, suffering, and anger often exist as illness strikes, aging advances, and people suffer losses, I have benefited from learning how individuals can temper their hardships with hope, peace, and humor.

One day, while I was reviewing my notes for this book, I was startled to realize that it had been many months since recording any new patient vignettes. During my 40-year career, rarely had a week passed without my jotting down a few memorable patient stories or quotes. Sadly, the challenge of the new burdensome documentation demands was interfering with my patient communication. These demands are focused on the diseases and the healthcare delivery process, not on the people. This does not seem like progress.

I began to wistfully apologize to my patients for spending so much time on the tasks that were disrupting our communication. Fortunately, the patients were forgiving as they were experiencing the same communication barriers with all their medical providers. Rather than accepting the situation, I used it as a wake-up call, resolving not to shortchange my patients. I stopped sacrificing valuable physician-patient encounter time to complete the new, expanded requirements of charting, billing, and coding, relegating these tasks to after-hours.

When the primary focus is on people, conversation occurs more naturally, allowing emotions to surface and humor to be expressed. Harvey Mackay writes about an Apache legend in which "the creator gave humans the ability to talk, to run, and to look at things. But in addition, the legend says he was not satisfied until he also gave them the ability to laugh. After giving humans this ability, the creator said, 'Now you are fit to live'" (2016).

Chapter 10

Lessons from Patients about Life, Work, and Family

"If you want to go fast, go alone; if you want to go far, go with others."

—*African proverb*

Whether in the office or in the hospital, a physician spends time diagnosing, testing, prescribing medications and therapy, encouraging lifestyle alterations, arranging surgery, and other referrals. However, it can be enlightening and enjoyable to encourage dialogue with patients, enabling them to teach us about their lives, work, and families.

Learning from Adults

Being a neurologist, I have found it useful to engage my patients in conversation unrelated to their medical issues. Besides establishing rapport, these free-ranging conversations have allowed me to evaluate their cognitive functioning, including their intelligence, judgment, knowledge, and experience.

Life: An unintended consequence of these conversations has been my ability to hear varied viewpoints about life. As illustrated by the following examples, some of these ring true, some do not, and others have unknown validity:

- A patient shared inherent wisdom by quoting an old African proverb, "The sun does not forget a village just because it is small."
- It often seems the case that "no one grows faster than the children of your friends, especially ones you see only occasionally."
- Whether valid or not, I laugh every time I recall a patient saying, "The answer is 'it's the money.' Now what was the question, doc?"
- Who can say whether a superstitious woman's belief is true that the "Devil's greatest trick is persuading people that he does not exist"?
- Certainly, it is unlikely to be true that "In Wisconsin, better eaters make better lovers."
- I hope it is not true that "The strongest thing about the weak is their hatred for the strong."

Work: To best understand my patients' histories, I routinely allowed time to discuss their occupational experiences. I relished hearing clever and sometimes fascinating descriptions of their work lives. One middle-aged woman, with a sour facial expression, said that she was "a happy hooker." When I looked rather surprised, she laughed, clarifying that she was a rug maker. Coincidentally, another patient worked at The Happy Hooker where she sold bait.

When I asked a man what he did at the Veterans Administration (VA) Hospital in Minneapolis, he responded, "Like everyone else at the VA, not much." On the other hand, some patients have high-stress jobs, contributing to their headaches, anxieties, and hypertension. One patient explained, "I work so much overtime, that about half the time I meet myself at work." In other words, he would still be at work when his next shift commenced.

A patient announced that he was "an observationalist" at work. While trying to clarify further, he promised me that he rarely got his hands dirty. Another generous and kind business consultant admitted that he was recently appointed to a nonprofit board of directors "because they could no longer afford my consultation fees but still wanted my input."

Family: An important part of the medical history is the family history. How wonderful to hear people who creatively describe their families:

- Sometimes they were serious: "My son is rudderless as he goes through life without direction."
- Sometimes they were clever: "I have two hands worth of children: six daughters, and four sons."
- Sometimes they were self-deprecating: "I have five children that own up to me."
- Sometimes they were silly: "We have four children. One of each kind."
- Sometimes they were humorously accurate: "I have three brothers and three sisters, so each of my sisters has four brothers."
- Sometimes they were sarcastic: "We have four children: three charming and active girls, and one vegetating teenage boy."

It is well known that a child's given name often has meaning and may influence a person's personality. One of my patients explained, "My mother knew that I would be gullible, so she named me Patsy." Another lovely, elderly woman, Antoinette, from a large Italian family, introduced me to her daughter, Toni. When I looked surprised, she clarified, "Yes, Toni was our youngest of nine children. We ran out of new names by the ninth, so we both share the same name."

Of course, not everyone has had children and not everyone marries:

- A 74-year-old widow explained that she had no children, because "I'm not ready yet."
- A never-married, single 84-year-old woman described herself as "an unclaimed pearl."
- A middle-aged woman introduced me to her long-term boyfriend, "I'm leasing him with an option to buy."
- Another woman came in with her boyfriend, whom I mistakenly referred to as her significant other. She corrected me promptly by saying that "he is not my significant other; I am the significant other."
- The long-term boyfriend of a patient quipped with a smirk, "We have been living in sin for 12 years, although there is precious little sinning going on these days."

Some of my patients are still looking for companionship, love, or possibly financial security. One woman admitted, "I will consider marrying any rich man with one foot in the grave and the other on a banana peel."

I have enjoyed hearing my patients describe their spouses and ex-spouses, their boyfriends and girlfriends. Their comments have provided insights into their lives and levels of happiness or stress at home. A happy woman gushed, "For years, I didn't realize that my husband was born to fetch." Another woman told me that the rumor is true, "If you marry them later in life, the husbands often come better trained." An elderly woman happily told me that she had "in life, achieved two wonderful husbands."

> ***"How should we like it were stars to burn with a passion for us we could not return? If equal affection cannot be, let the more loving one be me."***
> ***—W. H. Auden***

Some widows and widowers are lonely, but seem content to live alone with fond memories of their spouses. Many consider remarrying inconceivable. Some paint a picture of their deceased spouse as a saint, whether true or dramatically exaggerated.

An 88-year-old woman confessed to me that she would consider marrying again, if the man would promise three things: "First, he would take me wherever I wish. Second, he would not want any of that messing around in bed stuff. Third, my sister would also live with us." She did admit that, "I didn't know how spoiled I was."

In contrast to these widows, a few women marry multiple times. A nurse, who had been married three times, explained that "In life's competition to marry well-to-do widowers, nurses often get first choice."

One patient was a young, recent widow and rather lonely. She confided, "I miss the attention my husband would give me." She was even pleased to get a full-body patdown by a male TSA employee when her tight jeans with rhinestone bling set off the airport scanner.

An elderly widower complained to me that he missed his wife and her cooking. He was so inexperienced in the kitchen that his first attempt at cooking spaghetti was a disaster when it stuck to the empty pot after he boiled off all the water. Trying to rationalize his culinary disappointment, he explained: "The recipe said to boil the water before adding the spaghetti to the pot."

Hearing about my patients' marriages was both exhilarating and depressing. Some married couples stay together unhappily for many years for varied reasons. Some things I have been told casts doubt on the sanctity of some of their unions. One man confided in me that he "had never been on an airplane. The only times I have flown is when I made my wife really angry."

A senior citizen admitted that his recent marriage was not exactly what he was hoping for, as "I married Mrs. Wright, but only later learned that her first name was Always." Another patient described her husband as "reliably unreliable." A frustrated wife diagnosed her husband as suffering from "discretionary hearing."

An ironic situation occurred when a man complained that his wife refused to admit her hearing loss. We devised a plan to prove his case. After arriving home and hanging up his coat in the back hall, he planned to call out to his wife and ask what was for dinner. Hearing no response, he would then walk halfway to the kitchen, stop, and again ask what was for dinner. To demonstrate her hearing loss, he planned to walk up to her, kiss her, and ask a third time what was for dinner. After carrying out our plan, he lamented the result, as she had replied, "For the third time, honey, we are having roast beef."

When illness strikes a married couple, the healthy spouse responds in various ways. Some are wonderfully constituted to be caregivers. Many are kind and supportive. Some are not. Certainly, serious illness is stressful for all concerned. After a long illness leading to the demise of one spouse, the other spouse may also die shortly thereafter. The causes of the second death include loneliness, stress, and exhaustion or result from the caregiver having neglected her own health maintenance.

A husband who was exhausted caring for his wife's dramatic memory loss and personality change wondered if it was appropriate to "X-ray my wife's ass for a spring." She was constantly in useless motion. "If I convince her to relax and sit down, she pops up a second later as if she sat on a spring board."

It's well known that approximately half of all marriages end in divorce. These can be bitter, often leaving a person angry and spiteful. A 160-pound patient told me that, "Last year, I lost 180 pounds . . . I divorced him." Another woman was so angry after her divorce that she "would not even spit on him if he was on fire." Some are destined to repeat their mistakes. One patient suffered through five divorces. The only lesson she learned was that she would "never want to live with anyone again that eats or poops."

Of course, many married couples are happy. They have learned that once romantic love wanes, they remain fortunate to be married to a wonderful person. One likeable man put it this way: "My wife puts up with my bad habits, so I keep her watered and fed with plenty of sunshine." How bitterly sweet to hear an 81-year-old man lament, "I did not know what true happiness was till I married my second wife, who recently died. Sadly, we found each other too late."

It certainly seems hopeful for the institution of marriage when a man observes that his "43 years of marriage feels like a 43-year sleepover." Many marriages last because the participants adapt, evolve, and change. Long-term happiness often depends on flexibility, willingness to compromise, and embracing life with a sense of humor.

As one man told me, "I have learned that the husband is the head of the household, but the wife is the neck." Celebrating his long-standing marriage, an 80-year-old man's favorite toast was: "Here's to our ongoing happiness together, our decent health, and hoping neither of us has presenile dementia."

Making the right choices in life involves wisdom, experience, flexibility, an element of luck, and a good sense of humor. Choices that last are often based upon the ability to correctly gauge another person's worldview and their key personality characteristics, while realistically understanding their strengths and weaknesses. An insightful man put it this way: "Never laugh at your wife's choices; you were one of them."

With luck and insight, a person's experience brings the knowledge that not everything is of equal importance. Sometimes being right may be less important than living in harmony. My wife's grandfather was a wise man who taught her that relationships were the key to happiness: "When you win an argument, you may lose a friend." One patient wisely felt that "an apology does not necessarily mean you are wrong and the other person is right. It means that you appreciate the relationship more than who's right."

Learning and Working with Children and Teenagers

While I was not a pediatric neurologist, a significant portion of my neurology residency and three months of my rotating internship[38] were devoted to children. As I was comfortable with children once they were old enough to walk and talk, my professional life was enriched and diversified by including them in my practice.

Young children: I have marveled over the years at how charming children can be, while never knowing what they might say. After introducing myself and shaking hands with a five-year-old boy, he dutifully introduced his family, "This is my dad; that is my mom; and I'm the kid."

> *"A person's a person, no matter how small."*
> *—Dr. Seuss*

A four-year-old boy was brought to the clinic by his 84-year-old grandfather. The man could not wait to tell me that he had recently told his grandson how old he was. The young boy responded in awe, "Wow, Grandpa, did you start counting from one?"

For the very young, some of my questions to them were to access their cognitive abilities. Many of these were straightforward. For example, "Where is the sun at nighttime when it is dark?" However, some of my queries were unorthodox, yet effective and more fun:

- "Why did the man throw the clock out the window?" (Answer: He wanted to see time fly.)
- "Why did the same silly man sleep with a ruler?" (Answer: To see how long he slept.)

Because children can sometimes be shy and uncommunicative in a new doctor's office, the parents' interviews and school progress reports can be mined for facts about their brain development. A mother helped define her adorable but extraordinarily quiet six-year-old girl's intelligence by telling this story: "My daughter told me that she was going to draw a picture of God. When I told her that no one knows what God looks like, my daughter without hesitation said that everyone will know when I am done with my drawing."

---

[38] Rotating internships are rarely offered these days. My internship included rotations in multiple disciplines, including medicine, pediatrics, and obstetrics.

Some children are engaging, interactive, and talkative. I still smile when recalling a nine-year-old who asked me, "Don't you have any pills that don't taste like soap, doctor?"

Children can be concrete in their thinking, which can get other family members into trouble. An elderly woman admitted that her four-year-old grandson asked her husband to make the sound of a frog. When asked why, the boy responded, "Grandma told me that when you croaked, we could afford to go to Disney World."

Teenagers: Older children and teenagers can present unique challenges in the doctor's office. It should not be news that teenagers are a rather unique "species." They can be hilarious. For instance, a patient who found out she was pregnant asked her 16-year-old if he wanted a baby brother or baby sister. He responded, "I'd prefer a dog."

Teenagers can be sullen, withdrawn, and difficult to engage. Many have come to my office with a significant medical issue, like headaches, but must be prodded to tell their story, feeling safer avoiding interaction with an adult, especially a doctor. Even when forthcoming with their history, they are often guarded, steering clear of personal details as much as possible. I would never accept "I don't know" as an answer from a teenager, as it is usually an excuse to avoid an honest or thoughtful response.

It may indeed be difficult to get a meaningful history from a disengaged 16-year-old headache patient. Years ago, I discovered that brainteasers and riddles were helpful in engaging these young people by encouraging competitive responses. The riddles also served as a guide to judge their intelligence and their mood, while serving as useful surrogates to rather boring, "out-of-the-textbook" queries. Typically, the brainteasers also allowed me to observe an interaction between the patients and their parents, as they often struggled together to solve the puzzles.

I learned three riddles from my Uncle Ruby Leventhal when I was a teenager. I loved him dearly, was in awe of his keen wit and intelligence, and never forgot the lessons he taught me.

The first riddle was deceptively difficult:

> How many days does it take a spider to climb out of a 10-foot deep well? Each day, he climbs up one foot and, at night, he slides down exactly half a foot." The good math students would accurately calculate how many halves were in 10 and answer the riddle incorrectly by guessing, "20 days." (Answer: 19 days because the spider reaches the top of the well during the day #19, preventing him sliding back down half a foot that night)

A more straightforward but complicated-sounding math problem was also a favorite of Uncle Ruby's. While sounding dauntingly difficult to solve, the problem's answer can be revealed easily if a simple formula is utilized:

> Two cars start 60 miles apart and drive toward each other until they meet, each going 60 mph. How far would a fly fly, assuming the fly starts on the hood of one car and flies at 90 mph continually back and forth between the two cars as long as they are in motion. (Answer: 45 miles)

The third riddle was my favorite as Uncle Ruby created a brain teaser about two people's biological relationship:

> What is the relationship between two men if one remarks, "That man's father is my father's son; brothers and sisters I have none." For some inexplicable reason, the answer is obvious if the question is reversed and turned inside out. It would then read: "Brothers and sisters I have none (in other words, I am an only child); my father's son (me) is that man's father."

With good fortune, my initial consultation with a child or teenager would end with a reassurance to the parents that nothing was seriously wrong, typically followed by a three-part homework assignment:

1. Keep a detailed journal pertaining to the neurological issue, such as headaches or seizures.
2. Bring me a riddle to stump me next visit.
3. Bring the answer to a new puzzle I would typically introduce at the end of the consultation session, such as:

   Those who make them, do not want them. Those who buy them, do not use them. Those who use them, do not know it. What are they? (Answer: Coffins)

Summary

> *"We are all here on earth to help others; what on earth the others are here for I don't know."*
> *—W.H. Auden*

I have found that communicating with patients goes beyond taking the history of their medical problems, diagnosing their conditions, establishing a therapeutic plan, and counseling them as needed. To build rapport, gather diagnostic information, and ascertain the level of cognitive functioning, the clinician is helped by teasing out the details of a patient's family history, employment record, and worldview.

It is rarely emphasized that engaging in human dialogue with patients will also enrich the physician's life and decrease the chance of professional burnout. It is not a coincidence that burnout is at an all-time high as the system currently attempts to treat the physician-patient interaction as a business transaction, while deemphasizing the human side of medicine. I have been blessed with patients who have trusted me with their medical issues and concerns, while taking the time to educate me about life and family.

Chapter 11

The Wisdom of Patients Facing Aging and Death

"Death is the sound of distant thunder at a picnic."

—W. H. Auden

One of the challenging, yet rewarding aspects of being a neurologist is being a physician to the elderly. I have been intrigued by my time with our senior citizens. Whether immersed in a diagnostic dilemma, trying to improve their lives through treating a chronic malady, or just listening to their stories, I have learned a great deal about illness, aging, death, and dying.

A delightful woman summarized life nicely: "There are three stages of life: youth, middle age, and you look great."

As is well known and documented, public health measures and medical care advancements in the last century have resulted in an aging population. Many neurological conditions become more common with advancing age. Not having quick or easy fixes, these conditions ideally encourage seniors to develop effective coping skills.

Challenges to Diagnose and Treat the Elderly

Many unique challenges exist for any physician, but especially a neurologist when treating seniors. While the process of making a diagnosis should be similar for all patients no matter their age, the actual diagnoses can be more difficult to reach for the elderly.

> *"Old people have fewer diseases than the young, but their diseases never leave them."*
> *—Hippocrates*

Pre-existing, chronic conditions complicate diagnosis and treatment: To begin with, illnesses in the elderly usually do not occur in a vacuum, one at a time, as they do in the young and healthy. Pre-existing, chronic medical conditions, so common in the elderly, complicate medical care by:

- Increasing the difficulty of diagnosing new maladies.
- Decreasing the patient's ability to tolerate testing risks and complications.
- Changing the likelihood of new illnesses occurring.
- Making the treatment of new conditions at times more dangerous and possibly inappropriately useless.

Before launching into a new problem's differential diagnosis, the physician should consider the likely outcomes and ask questions, such as:

- Would the patient want and benefit from the identification of a new diagnosis?
- How well would treatment of a new diagnosis be tolerated?
- What are the chances of the treatment being successful?
- Would the patient authorize the treatment?

Balancing patient and family expectations and wishes: The formulation of a treatment plan must realistically take into account the patient's age, current status, and desires. The patient, the family, and the treatment team must all be "on the same page" when it comes to the patient's expectations and treatment options. At times, however, the expectations of the family and patient may be disparate, unrealistic, and/or inconsistent. This becomes especially problematic when the patient is in a medical crisis that interferes with his ability to clearly state his wishes and has not done so previously.

Terry Fulmer, president of the John A. Hartford Foundation, believes that "too many people with serious illness or at the end of life still receive care that's completely at odds with their own personal wishes" (Firth, 2016a). As she points out, Americans must expand the scope of meaningful discussions about end-of-life issues with their family and loved ones before their communities can decide fundamental life and death questions, including DNR (do not resuscitate), hospice, palliative care, and even assisted suicide and euthanasia (Firth, 2016a).

During a visit to my office, an elderly woman said, "Yes, I'm ready to die. As a matter of fact, I have already planned my fun-eral." "You mean your funeral," I responded. "No, doctor, I want everyone there to have fun and celebrate my life after I die! My will clearly details the funeral plans, including the location, the food to be served, the celebratory music to be played, and festive ambience for the entire day."

Living wills and family end-of-life discussions: For patients and their families in times of crisis, it is advantageous to prepare for end-of-life decisions. Aging patients need to identify a healthcare proxy, clarify their directives, and discuss end-of-life desires with their families and loved ones. These discussions may not be easy, but they are nonetheless incredibly valuable and comforting if and when a medical crisis occurs.

For example, what should be done if a situation seems *possibly* hopeless, but the doctors cannot give an absolute certain prognosis? What if the doctors say the situation is *probably* hopeless? Because even "miraculous recoveries" often leave the victim more impaired, what new disability would be acceptable to the patient and to what degree?

While important, formal living wills or advanced directives often fail to be definitively practical during medical emergencies when the ultimate prognosis is far from clear. They often specify the patient's instructions when definitive criteria exist, such as "if all hope is lost," or "if I will be in a permanent vegetative state." Such documents fail to satisfactorily clarify a person's wishes when the outcome of the medical crisis appears bleak, but cannot be considered definitely hopeless. It is best, therefore, for a living will to use the word "reasonable" when identifying situations in which patients request to be a DNR and/or a Comfort Care[39]. For example, "When it is reasonable to assume that all hope is lost."

It is not easy to predict what health crisis will occur or when difficult decisions will need to be made. We can, however, strive to have a realistic, up-to-date understanding of an elderly relative's quality of life. Is life becoming harder and harder? Is each day filled with more pain and less joy? Is memory failing with imminent institutionalization likely? Does Mom have something to live for? Family members should endeavor, for example, to understand clearly how an 85-year-old lives day-to-day with diabetes, congestive heart failure, arthritis, and memory loss.

In my experience, most elderly people fear lying in a hospital bed kept alive by machines, invasive tubes, and catheters more than they fear death itself. Yet, younger family members typically have more difficulty "giving up," allowing their elderly loved ones to die. During a medical crisis, family members of all ages must determine **what the patient would want,** not what they wish. In legalese, they should use "substituted judgment." The family must voice what course of action the ill person would choose in this circumstance, if he were competent.

Would he want to continue all care with the hope of recovering sufficiently to attend a wedding, see a grandchild grow up, read the next murder mystery, experience a Broadway play, witness a 400-pound tortoise walk in the Galapagos, enjoy the Minnesota Twins winning the next World Series, or finish a project like writing a memoir or knitting a blanket? Or will he likely be too ill and frail to enjoy life after this crisis, even if he beats the odds and survives?

A patient who describes herself as "on the sunny side of 80" may well want to be a "full code." This means she would want full resuscitation and all heroic medical treatments available. Another elderly woman who describes herself as "slowing down in every way possible" may indeed wish to be a DNR.

Physician end-of-life discussions: Unfortunately, many physicians are uncomfortable and often untrained to have end-of-life discussions with their patients. When polled, as many as half of the physicians have difficulty knowing what to say. In addition, even in the fields with the highest mortality rates, less than 30% of physicians have had formal training in addressing advanced care planning with their patients (Firth, 2016).

[39] Comfort care allows only treatment to relieve pain and suffering.

Besides life-or-death decisions, physicians have an important responsibility to discuss other end-of-life matters with their ill or dying patients, whether they are elderly or not. For a competent patient facing a new chronic and potentially fatal medical condition, a physician should ask four questions before embarking on the serious discussion of hospice:

1. What is your understanding of your health and disease? Especially in patients who have diseases that will likely cause them to die, it is paramount for the doctor to be convinced the patient and family both have a realistic understanding of the medical diagnosis and prognosis. This conversation often needs to occur more than once. It is typically insufficient, for example, for the patient and family to be told a single time that 90% of all patients with Lou Gehrig's disease die within three to five years. People hear and are ready to understand with clarity their diagnosis at different times and in different ways.

2. What are your goals if your health worsens? For example:

- Is the total number of days or months of life your number one concern?
- Is your main goal to have good quality time that is relatively pain-free?
- Are you willing to go through major complications of chemotherapy, radiation therapy, or surgery?
- How likely would the chance of improvement have to be to allow the possibility of such complications?
- Is there a specific event that you would like to be able to enjoy, like an upcoming wedding or a grandchild's birth?

3. What are your fears? For example:

- Do you fear death more than being disabled or sick?
- Do you fear for the people left behind without you?
- Do you fear "what is next"?
- Do you fear pain and treatment complications?
- Do you fear dying in the hospital alone?
- Do you fear putting your loved ones through the ordeal of your declining health?

- Do you fear not having the opportunity to say goodbye or finish a legacy project?

4. What tradeoffs are you willing to make that involve treatment options which come with risk of complications or pain? For the patient to answer this question, the physician must do a thorough presentation of the risks and benefits of treatment alternatives.

The 5 goodbyes: At some point, a physician's role evolves from being a diagnostic and treatment expert to counseling the patient and the family in how to best say goodbye. Neurologists "receive little formal palliative care training yet often need to discuss prognosis in serious illness, manage intractable symptoms in chronic progressive disease, and alleviate suffering for patients and their families" (Creutzfeldt, Robinson, & Holloway, 2016).

The physician should not abandon the patient when "all is lost." Unfortunately, I recall too often hearing a physician say, "There is nothing left to do for this patient." Even though it is easier to take this approach, as physicians we need to avoid this mentality. Indeed, I have fond memories of having provided significant comfort and counseling to patients and their families when there was "nothing else to do."

While the new field of palliative care is undoubtedly an advance, unfortunately it exists because many physicians limit themselves to attempting to cure disease, rather than accompany human beings through their illness. Discussing her new palliative care physician, a patient in a newspaper article exclaimed: "It was quite a relief. Our doctor listened to everything: the pain, the catheter, the vomiting, the tiredness. You can't bring up issues like this with an oncologist" (Span, 2016). In an ideal world where listening and counseling remain part of each physician's role, this new field would be unnecessary.

When death is imminent, I counsel families to follow the five-step process to say goodbye presented in page147. For this to be most effective, the patient and the family must be in similar stages of understanding, grief, and acceptance. When done right, saying goodbye can be beautiful and meaningful, facilitating a "good death," while bringing the family together emotionally to face death.

Slip-Sliding Away

Many elderly realize that they are failing:

- "Yup, this aging thing is catching up with me at 88 years old."
- "I'm old enough," a 93-year-old man told me when asked his age.
- "You don't have to ask, doctor. I'm a 79-year-old woman and I'm not so fine."
- "I have become psycho-ceramic; I'm like a cracked pot."
- "I have ODS: old duck syndrome."

Many know that the end is coming. It is not uncommon, as one 89-year-old woman told me, for people to open up the newspaper first to the obituaries to see if any of their friends have died: "As I'm now one of the moldy oldies, Dr. Schanfield."

Useful treatments and therapies exist for many chronic diseases that accompany advancing age, yet they are rarely cures. No treatment eliminates wear-and-tear degenerative arthritis and multiple other degenerative conditions, including neurological conditions of the brain, spine, and the peripheral nerves.

An elderly patient kept a positive attitude despite his difficulty walking caused by a combination of degenerative arthritis and a peripheral neuropathy.[40] Physical therapy treatment helped improve his gait, as it "was like a lube job for my knees and a flossing for the nerves."

Accompanying the aging process are mind and body disabilities, which commonly affect day-to-day living and the enjoyment of life. Some of my senior patients have expressed these issues in the following ways:

- "I'm becoming wimbly."
- "I am a LOL with OLL . . . a little, old lady with old-lady leakage."
- "I am falling so much now that it feels like, at times, I have only one gear and it is reverse."
- A frail, elderly man used 21st-century terms to describe his cognitive difficulties: "I can no longer multitask, as I have limited RAM."

---

[40] A peripheral neuropathy is a dysfunction of the nerves, usually in the hands and the feet, causing weakness, numbness, and pain.

A Migraine In Room 3, A Stroke In Room 4

Some of my elderly patients have variously described the evolution and deterioration of their bodies with endearing descriptions:

- An 86-year-old man told me that he had recently looked in the mirror and exclaimed, "How did we ever win World War II looking like that?"
- A 91-year-old tennis player, recognizing that he was slowing down, remarked, "Damn, at 90, I could have got to that ball."
- An active and relatively healthy 73-year-old widower described his new girlfriend to me by saying, "Unfortunately, she looks old, like me."
- An insightful man paused, smiled, and remarked, "The older I get, the better I was."

If we clearly listen to the elderly, they will often describe a life where the hardships of aging have overtaken the enjoyment:

- "I seem to have skipped the golden years and gone right to stainless steel."
- "The only thing golden is my urine these days."
- "I'm not sure if I'm rusting out or wearing out."
- "My mother is so thin that she now looks like a bicycle in storage with a sheet over it."

One evening, I was called to see a 92-year-old woman who suffered a cardiac arrest at home. Her 66-year-old son happened to arrive at her home as she collapsed, began resuscitation, and called 911. The paramedics arrived quickly and successfully restarted her arrested heartbeat. My hospital consultation on the night of admission found her unconscious with an uncertain prognosis. Remarkably, the next morning, I found her awake, fully recovered, and eating breakfast. I was still in her ICU room when her son rushed in, thrilled to find her recovered. However, the patient was not pleased and sternly scolded him, "At my age, you know I did not want to be resuscitated. If you ever do that to me again, I will haunt you for the rest of your life."

Besides being realistic as to their ultimate prognosis, some of the elderly long to maintain their dignity as they age. A 90-year-old woman was too embarrassed to call an ambulance when she fell and could not get up. Eventually, her neighbors convinced her to call for help. She reluctantly agreed to an ambulance, if it arrived with no lights flashing and no siren, and if the paramedics used the back door and back stairs of her apartment building.

Is it wrong to be elderly, in misery much of the time, and welcome death? A delightful 87-year-old woman with leukemia, severe arthritis, and seizures was only partially kidding when she asked, "I have a long life line, doctor. Can a person have that removed?"

In that same vein, a woman confided in me, "I'm ready. If there was an elevator button labeled 'Heaven,' I would push it." Unafraid of dying, a patient declared, "I am a DNR. Please remember that when I die, I would like cremation, as I look forward to being warm at least once in my life."

A dear man beautifully noted, "Death is something we all share, yet we can't share it with anyone."

I could not help but laugh when a man suggested, "My health situation now would make a monkey bite its mother." Putting this "had enough" philosophy in a worldly context, a thoughtful man confided in me that "the way the world is and the way I feel, I am glad that I am on the way out, rather than on the way in."

Chronic illness often leads a person to enjoy each day of life less. Not everyone is afraid of dying. Certainly, death is inevitable; sometimes it seems far off and sometimes close at hand. One day in the hospital, I came across an elderly, demented man watching the television intently, although it was not on.

Nursing Homes

In a bygone era, most of our senior citizens lived out their lives in their homes, surrounded and supported by their families. Today, many will end their lives in institutions, often nursing homes, doomed to an existence plagued with "boredom, loneliness, and helplessness" (Gawande, 2014). One of my patients described his nursing home as "a warehouse full of people waiting to die." However, dying at home can require significant resources and time, being realistically challenging and often impractical. Imagine the help needed to care for a 90-year-old widower with severe arthritis, incontinence, and dementia at home, when all his children work full-time.

Many of the nursing homes are underfunded and chronically understaffed, trying to provide adequate care for increasingly severely impaired and often demented patients. American nursing homes today serve as an important safety net, yet many have difficulty consistently providing 24-7 compassionate care. This has, at least in part, led to a new trend where families are feeling the need to covertly install spy-ware or granny-cams in nursing homes. Sadly, these families feel the need to surreptitiously record the nursing home care provided to forgetful seniors who cannot speak for themselves.

It is well known that social networks influence an individual's ability to function, especially when that individual is elderly. It is not a surprise that many seniors rapidly go "downhill" after being admitted to an institution with inadequate capacity to provide an active, engaging social milieu. While this may be the natural history of their condition, many at least partially fail because they are surrounded by people who are also failing physically and mentally. These institutions, like the hospitals, must strive to be more patient-centric, rather than focusing primarily on the organization of their processes and the needs of their staff.

A 97-year-old nursing home resident with delusions, paranoia, anxiety, and depression murdered her 100-year-old roommate in 2009 by placing a plastic bag over the roommate's head and pulling the covers over her. It took the deceased woman's family until 2016 to be granted a court hearing, attempting to hold the nursing home in Massachusetts accountable (Corkery & Silver-Greenberg, 2016). The delay was due to the nursing home in question, like many around the country, requiring all residents upon admission to sign a contract requiring binding arbitration should disputes arise.

This is concerning "because the secretive nature of arbitration can obscure patterns of wrongdoing from prospective residents and their families" (Corkery & Silver-Greenberg, 2016). In this case, "the arbitrator ruled in the nursing home's favor but provided no explanation. His ruling consisted of a single checkmark, indicating that (the nursing home) had not been negligent in its care." The patient's family later learned that the "arbitration firm running the hearing had previously handled more than 400 arbitrations for the law firm representing the nursing home company" (Corkery & Silver-Greenberg, 2016).

Our Healthy Seniors

Remarkably, in the 21st century, many of the elderly have their wits and their "marbles." Being relatively healthy, they are not institutionalized, but are aging at home independently. They have not been hospitalized numerous times nor are they in need of frequent, complicated clinic visits. One such vibrant and active 86-year-old patient said to me, "How dare they say that only the good die young?"

Some of us are indeed destined to live a long life. No one can argue that a man is doing well when he exclaims, "I'm 81 years old and still having fun." Some of our elderly are not ready to give up on life, despite their ailments and past medical issues. They can realistically laugh about aging:

- "I have asked you doctors to get me to 100, and I will take it from there."
- "Death wouldn't be so bad if it was not so darn permanent."
- "At my funeral, I want people to say, 'She was a wonderful person; she made the world a better place. Look, she's breathing!'"
- "I still got it, doc, I just don't know where I put it."
- A retired policeman joked that he is considering wearing a sign around his neck that reads, "Worn-out veteran, please do not discard."

Many of these cognitively intact senior citizens know who they are and what their priorities are. A lovely, 101-year-old woman, hospitalized for a small stroke, responded to questioning by exclaiming, "I'm left-handed. I'm red-headed. I'm nearsighted. I'm Catholic and I'd like to have communion."

> ***"I don't want to attain immortality through my work; I would prefer to attain it by not dying and living in my apartment."***
> ***—Woody Allen***

Many of our patients have interesting stories to tell. An elderly woman recalled losing consciousness, talking to dead relatives, and seeing a light at what appeared to be the end of a tunnel. She assumed she was dying. She then realized the light was dull; not bright as she had heard it described. She realized that she was not dying, but having a nightmare.

An elderly man was in a semi-conscious state in the ICU, near death for a number of days. While in "limbo," he recalled a conversation with his deceased brother in which they had made peace after an argument many years before. He remarkably recovered and awoke elated and at peace, as he had forgotten this reconciliation before the near-death experience.

Keys to Longevity

> *"Don't look back. Something might be gaining on you."*
> *—Satchel Paige*

In my career, I have often asked patients to share their secrets to a long life. Unquestionably, longevity hinges on heredity and a significant dose of good fortune. We all know, of course, that longevity often runs in families. For example, a patient remarked when I was taking his family history, "Neither of my parents died of anything serious in their 90s."

People with a family history of longevity may be nonchalant about death. As one man said, "My dad lost a courageous battle with longevity and died at 91 years old." When I asked the cause of death of a man's 95-year-old father, he remarked, "Doc, I didn't know a person needed a specific reason to die at 95."

It has been my privilege to have many witty and clever senior citizens as patients. One man unforgettably explained how to live a long life by saying, "Never spend a lot of time in a room that doesn't have a back door."

It is often not the number of years we spend on this mortal coil[41] that determines the quality and value of our lives. A long life may have little joy if not lived to the fullest. In contrast, a short life can be joyful, meaningful, and full of value. As Mae West famously remarked, "You only live once, but if you do it right, once is enough."

> *"Moderation in all things, especially moderation."*
> *—Ralph Waldo Emerson*

Some of my patients have stressed hard work, sweets, and alcohol in moderation as secrets to their longevity:

- An 84-year-old man was convinced that "the key to a long life is to have a large lawn that you cut yourself each week with a push mower."
- A patient, extolling the virtues of alcohol, described the key to a long life as "a double brandy and half a glass of beer each day."
- Sometimes the magic longevity formula included sweets, as an elderly woman confided in me: "A long life is generated and enhanced by a small piece of dark chocolate each day."

---

[41] The earth is referred to as a mortal coil in Shakespeare's "To be, or not to be" soliloquy in *Hamlet*.

- A witty 102-year-old man asserted that his "secret to a long life is two cocktails each day with regular exercise, especially if it is golf. I have even twice shot my age. Professional golfers can't say that."

Indeed, the role of work and exercise in longevity is suggested by recent animal research, which may apply to humans. Dr. John Krakauer's research suggests that exercise enhances brain function, increases the number of new brain cells, and increases myelination[42] of the neurons in an animal's motor cortexes. He postulates that "motor skills are as cognitively challenging in their way as traditional brainteasers" (Reynolds, 2016).

In addition to hard work, staying active seems crucial to living. Naomi Goldberg Haas has created a program to enroll older adults in dancing, because "movement enriches the quality of their lives. It's absolutely healing. Balance, mobility, strength—everything improves" (Brody, 2016). Besides activity itself, "social engagement has been repeatedly found in major population studies to prolong life and enhance healthy aging. Clinically, the programs have been linked to lower blood pressure, reduced levels of stress hormones, and increased levels of the happiness hormones that are responsible for a runner's high" (Brody, 2016).

Like many authors and researchers, I believe that being active, socially involved, and technologically connected avoids the isolation of aging. Colin Milner, the CEO of International Council on Active Aging, hypothesizes, "Being disconnected leads to isolation and depression." He predicts "by 2020, the second-leading cause of death globally would be depression, behind heart disease" (Gustke, 2016).

My elderly patients have also convinced me that attitude matters and is especially valuable when inherently positive. As a lovely 88-year-old recommended to me, "Enjoy every sandwich." This optimism seems to go hand-in-hand with longevity. Many have thrived by looking on the "bright side," often searching for the gift in a crisis. A 78-year-old, active man, who in retirement needed to earn additional income, smiled and told me, "I had to go back to work, so I took a job with 1,200 people under me. I cut the grass at a nearby cemetery."

Finding pleasure in the little things enhances the feeling of well-being in these optimistic people. Despite being relegated to institutional living, one man thanked

---

[42] Myelination is the process by which parts of a brain cell are insulated, so that the messages between neurons can proceed more quickly and smoothly.

his nursing home staff for painting the gray walls with bright and cheerful colors: "Thank heaven for the colorful paint on the walls. I was beginning to feel like I was living in a refrigerator."

A well-spoken, brilliant 84-year-old South American patient was a poet, who beautifully summarized for me her secret to a long, productive, and happy life: "La buena vida y el amor a tiempo." ("A good life and love at the right time.")

Dying with Warning

> *"A wise man ought to realize that health is his most valuable possession."*
> *—Hippocrates*

Of course, everyone dies. A few years ago, I was privileged to hear a series of amazingly insightful interviews of Dr. Bruce Kramer, the eloquent Dean of The School of Education at the University of St. Thomas, who later died after a multi-year battle with Amyotrophic Lateral Sclerosis[43] (Wurzer, 2011-2016). As his disease inexorably progressed and destroyed his muscles, he shared his journey publicly in print (Kramer & Wurzer, 2017) and online in a blog (Kramer, n.d.). He taught us the meaning of the phrase, "temporarily able-bodied" or, as he abbreviated it, "TAB." He reminded us that even when a person is in good health, it is only temporary, and surely not forever. Unless a person dies suddenly without pre-existing health problems, each of us will experience pain, disability, and illness.

Dr. Kramer understood that Americans typically feel embarrassed by the disabled people in their community. He identified a modern American myth that anyone should be able to overcome the ravages of physical or mental disability, if only they tried hard enough. Belief in this myth allows our society to justify the marginalization and isolation of the disabled and the dying among us, as if they are invisible. How sad and ironic that we tend to shun these neighbors, friends, and family in need, yet wish to be comforted and supported when we are struck down by disease and disability.

[43] Amyotrophic Lateral Sclerosis (ALS or Lou Gehrig's Disease) is a fatal neuromuscular disease.

Dying Young Without Warning

While longevity has become more common in America in the 21st century, many families still experience the premature loss of a loved one, often without warning. Sudden death in a young person eliminates the chance to say goodbye, while of course eliminating the person's ability to experience the fullness of the circle of life.

In a medical crisis, physicians' primary roles are to diagnose and institute appropriate treatment. As I have stressed throughout this book, physicians have an equally important role to communicate honestly with patients, family, and friends. As physicians, we can provide information about the medical crisis, eliminate blame, provide empathy, and respect the family's wishes. As physicians, we can only hope to initiate and aid in the grieving process. A family's attempt to cope with a loved one's life cut short by death is a long-term process, often accomplished with variable success.

My wonderful sister-in-law, Judy, died of a cerebral hemorrhage before turning 50. Her circle of life ended when her two daughters were 12 and 14 years old. She never experienced their making the cheerleading squad, excursions to buy prom dresses, their high school graduations, taking them to college, or planning a wedding. Dying young leaves a life unfinished.

Sadly, the sudden death of a young person eliminates the important human need to say goodbye, both for the patient and for the family. Those who loved my sister-in-law never got to say:

- I love you.
- I appreciate all you have taught me about life.
- I feel so fortunate to have had you in my life.
- I will miss you.
- I will make sure your daughters grow up to be good people and remember their mother.
- I promise that we will be okay, although it will not be easy without you.

When sudden death occurs, families typically never get to apologize, and say things like:

- "I forgive you for making me angry recently. I realize now that you were only trying to do what you thought was right."
- "I am sorry I yelled at you last week, Mom."

My sister-in-law was never able to tell her daughters, in a way they could understand as teenagers, how much they made her life meaningful, worthwhile, and complete. She was never able to tell her daughters what they meant to her and how important they were to her. She never had the opportunity to pass on to her daughters the important lessons of life and love she held dear. The opportunity for these most human of interactions between a parent and her children was lost forever.

My brother-in-law has embraced the choice to carry on and raise his daughters with abundant love and affection, thoughtfully and conscientiously placing them as the most important thing in his life. While he mastered the art of the barbeque, he had little time for embracing other culinary or domestic skills while being a single parent and president of a law firm. With little sleep, he has raised two wonderful young women to adulthood, while reminding them as best he could of their mother's values, hopes, and dreams.

Not all sons or daughters are as fortunate as my nieces. Their father accomplished an extraordinarily successful feat of raising them as a single parent. A physician friend of mine also lost his wife when their daughter was a teenager. Years later, he candidly discussed with me that life was a constant struggle raising his daughter by himself, while practicing medicine full-time.

Ten years after becoming a widower, his daughter angrily told him that he was often "not there" for her. Sad and apologetic, he pleaded with her to forgive him. He admitted that too often his goal was simply for the two of them to get through each day healthy, without a major crisis. After a long day working and functioning as a single parent, he sometimes had little energy left to do the "little things" that two parents can more easily accomplish.

Of course, it is trying, at times, to age with dignity as chronic medical conditions accumulate, interfering with the ability to enjoy life. Whenever possible, it is valuable to recall that death at a young age, especially without warning, is truly the most difficult thing for families to endure.

Summary

The practice of medicine that deals with aging, death, and dying can be especially challenging, yet I have found it often personally rewarding. The treatment of people as they die can be intellectually complex and emotionally exhausting. I have experienced such situations innumerable times, often finding them meaningful, embodying the essence of intimate human interaction.

> *"Age is a question of mind over matter. If you don't mind, it doesn't matter."*
> —*Satchel Paige*

My career has been grounded in listening. I am forever grateful to my patients for educating me about their lives, their wishes, their hopes, and their dreams. I am forever grateful to my patients for showing me how to cope with disease, disability, aging, and dying. I am forever grateful to my patients who have facilitated my learning the skills of palliative care.

When blessed with longevity, my patients have taught me what it means to "age gracefully." When death was imminent and a chance to say goodbye existed, hopefully my counsel helped them and their families cope and find some element of peace.

Mistakenly, our society, at times, seems to discount the elderly, making some senior citizens feel invisible. In my experience, many of our senior citizens are wise and witty, while being an invaluable resource to teach us how to live, cope with illness, and die. As one patient put it, "We have enough youth in America today. What we need to find now is a fountain of wisdom."

Part 4

WHAT'S NEXT?

As retirement approached, I interviewed multiple people about ways to give back to my community and my profession. Retirement has allowed me time to write, increase my teaching responsibilities, and enhance my connections with friends and family. I have little doubt that new ways to contribute to my community and my profession will present themselves.

The more vexing **Next Chapter** deals with the American healthcare system. It is my hope that this book will clarify the ills that have infected the current practice of medicine and lead to much-needed reforms.

Chapter 12

The Next Chapter

On October 1, 2015, I announced my retirement at the end of the year. This was not a snap decision. It was not caused by poor health, questions of competency, or production issues. It was time. It was my hope to retire before colleagues began to whisper questions concerning my practice proficiency, as I had witnessed with other colleagues. I wanted no crisis or malpractice event to cause my career to end with a "dud." I was fortunate to be able to retire on my own terms.

Reviewing my career by necessity has been intertwined with an analysis of changes in the American healthcare system. This final chapter therefore looks at what's next for me and for medicine.

Retirement

Retirement starts a new chapter of life, the beginning of a new way of living. I have been reminded that retirement is when you stop living at work and begin working at living.

One of my patients, Steve, described his retirement from a brilliant and demanding software development career as "going at 100 mph with my hair on fire to 0 mph." While I have, at times, felt like I was traveling at 100 mph with my hair on fire, my plan is not to downshift to 0 mph. My passion for patients and person-centered medical practice will not be retired. My passion during retirement will manifest itself in teaching, writing, and vigorously doing what I can to improve today's system of care.

Being fortunate to attain some level of success in life carries with it a responsibility to "send the elevator back down for the next person." Besides writing this book, I have chosen teaching as my preferred method of giving back. I have been asked to continue tutoring and lecturing the medical students at the University of Minnesota in the Department of Neurology, and hope to expand my presence there. I have also volunteered to mentor family practice medical residents who serve the underprivileged in St. Paul. In addition, I will serve on committees to improve nursing home care and to upgrade Native American epilepsy care.

"It had long since come to my attention that people of accomplishment rarely sat back and let things happen to them. They went out and happened to things."
—Leonardo da Vinci.

Stepping away from Neurological Associates of St. Paul: Without question, I will miss working at Neurological Associates of St. Paul. By the end of 2015, the time had come to move on to the next chapter of life. It was time for the younger physicians to "step up to the plate." It was appropriate to allow other physicians in our group to carry the burden of adjusting to the rapidly changing environment. It was time for others to run Neurological Associates of St. Paul, a small business in an increasingly regulated industry with proliferating insurance "red tape" and government oversight. It was time to get off the treadmill of seeing ever-increasing numbers of clinic and hospital patients to try to stay ahead of the accelerating rate of overhead expenses.

Beginning in 2013, I began to take limited "on call" responsibility. I worked the same number of "call nights" each year, but avoided working overnight, weekends, and holiday shifts. These changes facilitated a smoother transition, while keeping me fresh to practice medicine as I believed appropriate.

I will miss the camaraderie of working with my partners, nurses, and staff. For 38 years, we were blessed with minimal staff turnover, leading to long-term working relationships. The first nurse we hired in 1978, Andrea, retired about the same time I did, marking her hiring as one of our best decisions. Patty, the clinic nurse who worked with me the most, was a blessing, being keenly intelligent, knowledgeable, hardworking, kind, and caring. Practicing medicine without her help would have been infinitely more difficult.

Every person employed in a medical office has an important and unique role. The first person a patient interacts with is often the telephone operator. Gail, our dedicated and conscientious telephone operator, faithfully paged me every day with my daily calendar and other reminders. I smile every time I recall this page from Gail: "It's national doughnut day, Dr. Schanfield, and we have no doughnuts in the office."

Our medical secretaries typically spent a significant portion of each day answering the phones. During a busy clinic day, Stacy, one our efficient, savvy secretaries, once answered the phone in a way I will never forget. While looking at a picture of her son, she picked up the phone and asked, "How may I love you today?"

Each of my partners had a unique personality and style, yet we all blended together cohesively in our small group practice. Early in his career, my partner, Dr. Peter Boardman, announced humbly and humorously, "It is once again time to play help the new guy." His memorable witticisms continued long after he was no longer the "new guy," such as his acerbic pronouncement: "It is my weekend to celebrate the institution of being on call."

Dr. Boardman, a philosophy major in college, wrote exceptionally vivid, memorable chart notes, choosing not to follow the practice of generic, bland documentations. Once, he chose to state his opinion that his patient would soon die by writing, "She will not be on this mortal coil[44] much longer." For another thriving patient, he recorded the "patient's strength as six on a five-point scale."

I recall Dr. Boardman being asked to see an agitated, hostile, and confused hospital patient. He documented that his plan was "to order testing for the usual suspects that cause delirium." A few days later, he wrote the following hospital note:

> The patient remains belligerent and swears frequently; today, though, he lacks his previous flair in his choice of negative comments, which diminishes the entertainment factor in today's hospital encounter. In addition, I should note that the patient also did not find my hospital visit with him compelling nor interesting.

---

[44] As I noted earlier, the earth is referred to as a mortal coil in Shakespeare's "To be, or not to be" soliloquy in *Hamlet.*

Patients say goodbye: Because I announced my retirement three months in advance, the transition was more meaningful and emotional than I anticipated. Each day, I experienced multiple people (patients, nurses, staff, doctors, hospital administrators, secretaries, and technicians) wishing me well and saying goodbye, sometimes in memorable ways. During her final office visit, a female patient smiled and complained, "Oh, I hate breaking in new men."

A 62-year-old patient brought his wife for our final visit. We first discussed his multifocal motor neuropathy[45] that had initially threatened his ability to walk, but had been well controlled for years on twice-a-month infusion treatments. After the medical follow-up portion of the office visit, the patient, bubbling with visible excitement, handed me an envelope. Inside the envelope was a job application filled out with my name, age, and current work address. The application was for a job as a "carry out" person at a Trader Joe's grocery store to start after the first of the year. On the line that asked for the applicant's last job's salary, he had typed in "None of your business." As I read this document out loud, we all howled with laughter.

Certainly, it is common for patients to bond with their physicians and be ambivalent when they retire. This results in many bittersweet goodbyes:

- "It's hard to believe that it was 18 years ago that I met you and you diagnosed me correctly, after struggling with a variety of symptoms for nine months. Although it was not what someone wants to be told: 'You have this and there is no cure.' As I told you recently, at least one good thing came out of it, knowing you and your nurse, Patty. It is so strange to think that you will be starting a whole new, different life. I'm very happy for you, but I will sure miss the sense of security I've felt all these years knowing you were there. I guess it's only fair you retire. From my perspective, you fulfilled what you promised me. When diagnosed in 1997, I asked you to please help me to be OK until my little boy was grown up. He's now 27 and married, so I think you actually did better than keep your promise."
- "From the moment you blew into my hospital room over a year ago and diagnosed me, medicated me, and got me out of that hospital the next day, you have been our hero. We so hate to see you go, but we are also so happy for you. We hope your life is filled with health, happiness, and lots of fun,

---

[45] A multifocal motor neuropathy is an autoimmune inflammation of the myelin of the peripheral nerves, which this man had successfully treated by periodic intravenous gamma globulin infusions, composed of processed plasma containing other people's antibodies.

as you so deserve it. Be safe in your travels and may God bless and watch over you."

- "Hi, Dr. Schanfield. I want you to know that I appreciated your care and liked being your patient. From the first appointment to the last, you always made me feel good about myself, despite the Parkinson's. The Parkinson's has brought changes, but they haven't been drastic. Thanks for encouraging me! This kooky card of an orangutan saying 'Thanks' just seemed to fit. I don't quite know why, but I giggled and said, 'That's it.' May your retirement years be many and filled with joy and laughter. I pray that God will bless you and your family as you experience your new lifestyle."
- "I just wanted to take this time to thank you for 15 years of your caring and kind medical care. It started when you diagnosed my MS. I knew nothing about the illness. You have seen me through numbness, tingling, shingles, cognitive issues, optic neuritis, sleeplessness, and work issues. But for all of that, I am still walking and working; best of all, I'm playing with my granddaughters! So thank you for making it all happen. I am going to miss you. Congratulations on your retirement."

Claudia, a lovely stroke patient, brought tears to my eyes while reading her note:

> "Thank you for being my neurologist. You care, not only for my brain, but also for me as a person—the 'thing' that makes me me! You never let me settle for less than the best I could do. So I climbed Carlton Peak; I kayaked on Lake Superior; I do Eagle Pose in yoga; I do stand-up paddle boarding; I play on the floor and in the trees with my granddaughter; I try new things. Best wishes in the days and years ahead!"

Claudia is correct. I have tried to encourage my patients "to do." I have routinely pushed my patients to be as active as physically possible and not allow their medical conditions or their age to define them. I believe a follow-up office evaluation after a stroke, such as the one Claudia suffered, is not limited to reviewing blood pressure, diet, cholesterol, and medications, while searching for signs of a new stroke. A complete visit incorporates how the patient feels and functions day-to-day, week-to-week, and month-to-month.

A final, unexpected card came from a patient's wife. Years before, the patient had suffered a catastrophic head injury for which we could do very little:

> "I heard that you will be retiring soon, and I want to take this moment to say thank you for the wonderful care you gave my husband, James. I was so blessed to have met you during the worst time in my life, after my husband

> suffered his brain injury. Enjoy your retirement and here's wishing you the very best retirement and next phase in life! Have a glass of vino on me."

Colleagues say goodbye: Besides benefiting from our terrific staff and being blessed with wonderful patients, my colleagues in all fields of medicine have enhanced my professional life. Out of necessity, neurosurgeons and neurologists work closely together and I have been blessed to work with some of the best.

The increase in certified nurse practitioner (CNP) utilization has been especially helpful in neurosurgery. Because neurosurgery operations can be unpredictably prolonged, CNPs appropriately fill the neurosurgical communication role with patients, families, and fellow practitioners, including neurologists.

It was especially difficult for me to say goodbye to Katie and Sherilyn, two bright and conscientious neurosurgical nurse practitioners, whom I first met when they were ICU nurses. I will long remember a retirement card from Sherilyn, who wrote, "When I heard of your retirement, it left a little hole in my heart. I will miss your wisdom and sense of humor."

As we go through life doing what we do, we seldom understand the impact we have on others. Besides spending countless hours teaching medical students and medical residents, it has been my pleasure to also mentor young people considering medicine. Samantha, a premed student who "shadowed" me for a year, handed me a lovely thank you card:

> Thank you for your guidance.
> Thank you for your mentorship.
> Thank you for your time and humor and your kindness.
> Thank you for your support.
> Most importantly, thank you for your friendship.

Memories of physician colleagues: I will miss chatting with other physicians in the doctor's lounge and sharing a lifetime of "war stories" and occasional lapses into gallows humor. My surgical colleagues' remarks included:

- "In the operating room, *'oops'* is a four letter word."
- "Minor surgery is any surgery done on somebody other than the surgeon and her family."
- "Minor surgical complication means the surgeon has no need to explain."

- "Major surgical complication means the physician had better explain."
- Orthopedic surgery by necessity attracts the physically strong and mechanically inclined. The joke is that "the most difficult training period for an orthopedic surgeon is the second time through fourth grade."

My obstetrical colleagues' war stories included:

- A man called his wife's obstetrician at 3:00 a.m. and asked how to deliver kittens.
- A patient called her obstetrician on Sunday morning at 7:00 a.m. to ask, "Can I have sex this morning? I am scheduled to have artificial insemination on Monday."

Medical diagnoses can be difficult, resulting in one physician describing his uncertainty as "analysis paralysis." Another colleague defined an interesting patient case: "Don't know the diagnosis; don't know the correct treatment; fortunately he is not my patient."

Medicine has provided me a life of professional challenges and rewards. Most of all, I am grateful for the people, including my patients, colleagues, and staff.

What's Next for Healthcare in America?

In 2009, Dr. Stephen Sergay, president of the American Academy of Neurology, led a call for a significant change in our healthcare system:

> Physicians must rescue our medical profession and professionalism as care-givers, not as providers of a commodity through "encounters" and tests, but as practitioners who engage in human interactions, often responding to the needs of ill or frightened human beings. Our patients are not just "lives" or "customers"; healthcare reform will fail unless it is organized around the patient-doctor relationship. . . . We must come together morally, not by self-interest. We are being manipulated without consideration for our ethos nor our historical patient-doctor contract. . . . Science complexity is rapidly increasing, as are the needs for specialization

> ***"The bottom line: healthcare reform is about the patient, not about the physician."***
> ***—Abraham Verghese***

> and subspecialization. The center of our healthcare system must rest on the ancient physician-patient contract, with personal responsibility on the part of the physician and the patient. (Sergay, 2009, p. 1235)

A recent survey lent support to Dr. Sergay's views, as three-quarters of medical students, residents, and physicians identified "helping people" as the key to their pursuing medicine (Saint Jacques, 2017). Unfortunately, for every patient care hour, a physician now spends a minimum of two hours on bookkeeping and other tasks, interfering with the fulfillment of physician professional expectations (Busis, 2017).

In other words, today's physician spends much less time in direct patient care than ever before. Time interacting with patients has been replaced by hours of EMR and other desk work tasks. These tasks include clerical documentation, electronic medical record updates, protocol management, medical prior authorizations, audits, and other oversight requirements. This changing work pattern certainly diminished my feeling of accomplishment and enjoyment.

This does not have to be the case. For example, Dr. Michael Neren postulates that the EMR can be materially "humanized," simply by including sections on the establishment of patient rapport.

Previous U.S. Health and Human Services Secretary Dr. Tom Price agrees that the goal should be to "collect data on physician performance without inundating doctors and nurses and administrators with costly, time-consuming paperwork . . . We've turned a lot of folks in the healthcare professions into data entry clerks" (Clark, 2017).

While writing and researching this book, the facts confirmed what I had suspected. Burnout is a major current crisis amongst physicians, including neurologists. Sixty percent of neurologists report burnout symptoms, including high emotional exhaustion and depersonalization (Owens, 2017). Was this phenomenon a factor in my decision to retire? My decision was certainly influenced by changes in the profession that directly contribute to the burnout crisis.

My primary reason for being a clinician was to interact with people in need. Accomplishing this goal justified the demanding and grueling 60- to 70-hour workweeks, including numerous "on call" hours spent at night, on weekends, and holidays, away from family and friends. For much of my career, the time spent was worthwhile.

If our healthcare system in America is to be improved, the physician-patient contract, as spelled out by the Hippocratic Oath, must be enhanced. It is my hope that this enhancement would include instituting the following suggestions, emphasized in this book:

1. **Treat human beings:** Encourage physicians to treat human beings in need instead of treating health problems, such as "a migraine in room #3; a stroke in room #4." Patient-centric care must be at the center of our system, rather than the current primary focus on the system and the providers.
2. **Emphasize physician social-emotional skills**: Formally incorporate the education of social-emotional skills, including listening and communication; empathy, honesty, humility, and rapport building; and the counseling of patients.
3. **Increase meaningful physician-patient face time:** Facilitate an increase in available time and resources for direct, long-term physician-patient interaction. This should include returning "your physician" to the bedside in the hospital as well as the clinic.
4. **Strengthen collaboration:** The physician-patient partnership should be enhanced by emphasizing active patient involvement and shared decision-making, while requiring reasonable patient compliance and durable lifestyle alterations.
5. **Decrease healthcare fragmentation:** Enhance communication among physicians and all components of the healthcare system to improve the patient's well-being and ability to navigate the system.
6. **Ease the burden of record keeping:** Humanize and increase the efficiency of the EMR, while reassigning much of the current physician and nursing documentation and paperwork to qualified support staff.
7. **Ensure judicious utilization of physician extenders:** Educate clinicians in the utilization and oversight of physician extenders.
8. **Improve general residency training programs:** Require all medical and surgical residencies to be more comprehensive so as to decrease the need for potentially dehumanizing subspecialty fellowships.
9. **Adjust the number of physicians trained:** Base the number and fields of physicians trained more directly on the needs of the served patient population.
10. **Emphasize the whole body, proactive care model:** Demand that our healthcare system be based on best practice in a coordinated, proactive approach that takes into account a person's lifetime wishes and goals for their

entire body; recognize that an episodic care model, which deals with isolated problems, is but one important component of best practice.

This book opened with the assertion that healthcare in America is in crisis. I hope this publication clarifies, at least in some small way, many of the fundamental ills currently infecting our system of care, while advancing the discussion of a successful prescription for improvement. It is of paramount importance to focus primarily on the needs of the patients. It is essential that the emphasis be shifted back to listening to patients, while treating them as human beings in need. I may not have all the answers. Fortunately, many brilliant minds are working diligently to enhance and upgrade the healthcare system to bring it back into balance. It is my hope that those with the power to improve our system will listen and take appropriate action in the near future.

REFERENCES

2015 state physician workforce data book. (2015). Association of American Medical Colleges. Retrieved from https://www.aamc.org/data/workforce/reports/442830/statedataandreports.html

American Medical Association. (2017, March 30). Survey: *U.S. physicians overwhelmingly satisfied with career choice* [Press release]. Retrieved from https://www.ama-assn.org/survey-us-physicians-overwhelmingly-satisfied-career-choice

Avitzur, O. (2016, April/May). Boost brain health: Try these science-backed (and affordable) strategies to preserve and protect your brain. *Neurology Now, 12*(2), 6.

Baker, A. (1958). *An outline of clinical neurology.* Dubuque, Iowa: William C. Brown Book Company.

Belluck, P. (2016, February 10). Education may cut dementia risk, study finds. *The New York Times.* Retrieved from https://www.nytimes.com/2016/02/11/health/education-may-cut-dementia-risk-study-finds.html

Bernard, D. (2012, March 23). The baby boomer number game. *U.S. News & World Report.* Retrieved from https://money.usnews.com/money/blogs/on-retirement/2012/03/23/the-baby-boomer-number-game

Brody, J. E. (2016, March 7). Using the arts to promote healthy aging. *The New York Times.* Retrieved from https://well.blogs.nytimes.com/2016/03/07/using-the-arts-to-promote-healthy-aging/

Brooks, M. (2016, May 5). US medical school enrollment up 25% since 2002. *Medscape.* Retrieved from http://www.medscape.com/viewarticle/862956

Buettner, D. (2008). *The blue zones.* Des Moines, IA: National Geographic.

Busis, N. (2017, January 19). Best advances of 2016 in Practice Management/Professionalism. *Neurology Today, 17*(2): 30.

Cameron, W. B. (1963). *Informal sociology: A casual introduction to sociological thinking.* New York: Random House.

Casarett, D. (2016, March 31). The science of choosing wisely —- Overcoming the therapeutic illusion. *The New England Journal of Medicine, 374,* 1203-1205.

Chen, P. W. (2013, May 30). For new doctors, 8 minutes per patient. *The New York Times.* Retrieved from https://well.blogs.nytimes.com/2013/05/30/for-new-doctors-8-minutes-per-patient/?_r=1.

Clark, C. (2016, March 28). 10 ways EHRs lead to burnout. *Family Practice News.* Retrieved from http://www.mdedge.com/familypracticenews/article/107632/practice-management/10-ways-ehrs-lead-burnout

Clark, C. (2016, April 15). Dell Medical School: A unique agenda for a new era. *Hospitalist News: News and Views that Matter to Physicians.*

Clark, C. (2017, June 26). Secy. Price: HHS won't dictate to docs — Promises flexibility in pushing value-based payment; fee-for-service may remain for some situations. *MedPage Today.* Retrieved from https://www.medpagetoday.com/PublicHealthPolicy/HealthPolicy/66262

Corkery, M. & Silver-Greenberg, J. (2016, February 21). Pivotal nursing home suite raises a simple question: Who signed the contract? *The New York Times.* Retrieved from https://www.nytimes.com/2016/02/22/business/dealbook/pivotal-nursing-home-suit-raises-a-simple-question-who-signed-the-contract.html

Creutzfeldt, C. J., Robinson, M. T., & Holloway, R. G. (2016, February). Neurologists as primary palliative care providers: Communication and practice approaches. *Neurology: Clinical Practice, 6*(1), 40-48.

Dark chocolate found to offer brain health benefits. (2015, November/December). *Practical Neurology, 15*(6).

Day, G. S. (2016, September). Symptomatic management of dementia. *Neurology Reviews, 24*(9),16, 21.

Dominick, P. (2017, July 3). Aspen Ideas Festival: The social downside to technology. *Minnesota Public Radio News.* Retrieved from https://www.mprnews.org/story/2017/07/03/aspen-ideas-the-social-downside-to-technology

Dorsey, E. R. (2016, February). Editorial: Silent majority. *Neurology: Clinical Practice, 6*(1), 11.

Drummond, D. (n.d.). I don't always get sucked into a jet engine but when I do, I use ICD-10: V97.33XD meme. *The Happy MD.* Retrieved from https://www.thehappymd.com/blog/icd-10-and-the-most-interesting-man-in-the-world

Dykes, D. & Chase, J. (2016, October). Evaluating surgical outcomes. *Minnesota Physician, XXX*(7), 32-34.

Dylan, B. (1963). The times they are a-changin'. *The times they are a-changin'.* Burbank, CA: Warner Bros, Inc.

Fallik, D. (2016, February). When a hospital threatened to outsource their services, a team of hospitalists unionized: Neurohospitalists say they can relate to similar pressures. *Neurology Today, 16*(4), 28, 33.

Fallik, D. (2016, February 18). Diagnostic errors are a 'blindspot' in medicine: The most common mistakes in neurology, and why they occur. *Neurology Today, 16*(5), 8-9.

Federal Trade Commission. (2016, January 5). *Lumosity to pay $2 million to settle FTC deceptive advertising charges for its "brain training" program* [Press release]. Retrieved from https://www.ftc.gov/news-events/press-releases/2016/01/lumosity-pay-2-million-settle-ftc-deceptive-advertising-charges

Fiore, K. (2016, April 13). Opioid crisis: Scrap pain as 5th vital sign? *MedPage Today.* Retrieved from https://www.medpagetoday.com/publichealthpolicy/publichealth/57336

Firth, S. (2016, April 15). Docs still flinching on advanced care planning — Survey explores barriers to talking to patients about end-of-life decisions. *MedPage Today.* Retrieved from http://www.medpagetoday.com/publichealthpolicy/generalprofessionalissues/57375

Firth, S. (2016, April 27). 10 questions: Leana Wen, MD — Health commissioner and ER physician says most of what impacts patient's health happens outside the hospital. *MedPage Today.* Retrieved from http://www.medpagetoday.com/Blogs/10Questions/57562

Fitzgerald, S. (2016, March). Seafood found neuroprotective for Alzheimer's in those with risk gene. *Neurology Today, 16*(5), 1, 5-8.

Frieden, J. (2016, April 16). D.C. week: CMS announces new model for primary care — Advisory committee recommends FDA delay approval for a new EGFR inhibitor. *MedPage Today.* Retrieved from https://www.medpagetoday.com/washington-watch/washington-watch/57391

Gardner, H. (1993). *Frames of mind: The theory of multiple intelligences* (10th ed.). New York: Basic Books.

Gawande, A. (2014). *Being mortal: Medicine and what matters in the end.* Waterville, ME: Thorndike Press.

Goldenberg, J. M. (2016, February). The breadth and burden of data collection in clinical practice. *Neurology: Clinical Practice, 6*(1), 81-86.

Grau, J. (2016, April 21). *Why quality?* [Video webinar]. Sponsored by the National Quality Forum.

Greb, E. (2016, September). Modifiable factors may protect memory despite genetic risk for Alzheimer's Disease. *Neurology Reviews, 24*(9), 14.

Gustke, C. (2016, March 11). Making technology easier for older people to use. The New York Times. Retrieved from https://www.nytimes.com/2016/03/12/your-money/making-technology-easier-for-older-people-to-use.html

Hawton, M. (2016, March). Health literacy: Creating a better-informed patient. *Minnesota Physician, XXIX*(12), 26-27.

Herman, A. E. (2016). *Visual intelligence: Sharpen your perception, change your life.* New York: Eamon Dolan Books, 188.

Hewitt, J. (2017, February 2017). How to grow old like an athlete. *World Economic Forum.* Retrieved from https://www.weforum.org/agenda/2017/02/healthspan-vs-lifespan/

Jena, A. B. (2015, November 4). Physician spending and subsequent risk of malpractice claims: observational study. *The BMJ, 351,* h5516. Retrieved from http://www.bmj.com/content/351/bmj.h5516

Johnson, C. (2016, February). Dying from prescription heroin: A perspective on the opiate epidemic. *Minnesota Physician, XXIX*(11), 30-32.

Johnson, T. A. & Marcotte, J. C. (2016, February). Electronic health record systems: Choices, challenges, and dollar signs. *Minnesota Physician, XXIX*(11), 34-36.

Joshi, N. (2015, January 4). The opinion pages: Doctor, shut up and listen. *The New York Times.* Retrieved from https://www.nytimes.com/2015/01/05/opinion/doctor-shut-up-and-listen.html

Kalanithi, P. (2016). *When breath becomes air.* New York: Random House, 166.

Keaten, J. (2016, April 6). WHO: Diabetes rises fourfold over last quarter-century. *The Associated Press.* Retrieved from https://apnews.com/c575f45cdcc340e5a68c61c3aec85eb5/who-diabetes-rises-fourfold-over-last-quarter-century

Kieran, K. (2016, March). Breaking bad news: A challenge we all face. *Minnesota Physician, XXIX*(12), 28-29, 38.

Kolata, G. (2016, December 12). One weight-loss approach fits all? No, not even close. *The New York Times.* Retrieved from https://www.nytimes.com/2016/12/12/health/weight-loss-obesity.html

Kramer, B. H. (n.d.). *Dis Ease Diary.* Retrieved from http://diseasediary.wordpress.com

Kramer, B. H. & Wurzer, C. (2017). *We know how this ends: Living while dying.* Minneapolis,

MN: University of Minnesota Press.

Kübler-Ross, E. (1969). *On death and dying.* London: Routledge.

Lasagna, L. (1964). A modern Hippocratic Oath. *Association of American Physicians and Surgeons, Inc.* Retrieved from http://www.aapsonline.org/ethics/oaths.htm#lasagna

Levine, J. A. (2002, December 16). Non-exercise activity thermogenesis (NEAT), a review article. *Best Practice & Research: Clinical Endocrinology & Metabolism, 16*(4), 679-702.

Lipska, B. K. (2016, March 12). The neuroscientist who lost her mind. *The New York Times.* Retrieved from https://www.nytimes.com/2016/03/13/opinion/sunday/the-neuroscientist-who-lost-her-mind.html

Mackay, H. (2016, April 3). In business and life, a sense of humor helps. *Star Tribune.* Retrieved from http://www.startribune.com/in-business-and-life-a-sense-of-humor-helps/374331251/

Marshall, P. (Director). (1990) *Awakening*s [Motion picture]. Columbia Pictures.

Moon, M. (2016, April 13). Benefit of lumbar fusion for spinal stenosis found to be small to nonexistent. *Clinical Neurology News.*

Moore, G. (2013, January 11). RAND Corp. backs off GE-funded study, finds few savings in electronic medical records. *Boston Business Journal.* Retrieved from https://www.bizjournals.com/boston/blog/mass_roundup/2013/01/emr-savings.html

Morris, M. C., Brockman, J., Schneider, J. A., Wang, Y., Bennett, D. A., Tangney, C. C., & van de Rest, O. (2016, February). Association of seafood consumption, brain mercury level, and APOE e4 status with brain neuropathology in older adults. *JAMA, 315*(5), 489-497.

Murphy, D. R., Meyer, A. N. D., Russo, E., Sittig, D. F., Wei, L., & Singh, H. (2016, April). The burden of inbox notifications in commercial electronic health records. *JAMA International Medicine, 176*(4), 559-560.

Ohno, T. (2006, March). Ask 'why' five times about every matter. *Toyota Traditions, Toyota.* Retrieved from http://www.toyota-global.com/company/toyota_traditions/quality/mar_apr_2006.html

Olson, J. (2015, September 19). Health beat: Misdiagnosis solutions generated by St. Paul think tank. *Star Tribune.* Retrieved from http://m.startribune.com//health-beat-misdiagnosis-solutions-generated-by-st-paul-think-tank/328348461/

Olson, J. (2016, January 27). Chronically ill Minnesota patients eight times more expensive than healthy patients. *Star Tribune.* Retrieved from http://www.startribune.com/chronically-ill-patients-eight-times-more-expensive-than-healthy-patients/366649711/

Over-70s only! Manchester opens playground for oldies. (2008, January 30). *The Guardian*. Retrieved from https://www.theguardian.com/uk/2008/jan/30/society.healthandwellbeing

Owens, S. (2017, March 16). AAN survey: Six out of ten neurologists report felling burned out: What can be done to fix the problem? *Neurology Today, 17*(6), 16-19.

Paddock, C. (2010, January 21). Life's simple 7 measures for healthy heart. *Medical News Today*. Retrieved from http://www.medicalnewstoday.com/articles/176651.php

Parkinson, J. (1817). *An essay on the shaking palsy*. London: Whittingham and Rowland for Sherwood, Neely, and Jones.

Peckel, L. (2016, February). Modifiable risk factors for Alzheimer's Disease point to preventive strategies. *Neurology Reviews, 24*(2), 18-19.

Pheifer, P. & Walsh, P. (2015, September 13). 90-year-old who fatally shot son in Maplewood said to have Alzheimer's. *Star Tribune*. Retrieved from http://www.startribune.com/90-year-old-fatally-shoots-son-in-maplewood-home-calls-911-and-waits-for-police/327182641/

Reynolds, G. (2016, March 2). Learning a new sport may be good for the brain. *The New York Times*. Retrieved from https://well.blogs.nytimes.com/2016/03/02/learning-a-new-sport-may-be-good-for-the-brain/

Robinson, E. (2016, September). How are migraine and stress related? *Neurology Reviews, 24*(9), 8.

Robinson, E. (2016, October). Mentally stimulating lifestyle may protect cognition from the effects of a poor diet. *Neurology Reviews, 24*(10), 38.

Rothschild Levi, J. (2016, March 15). Humor me, heal me. *The Times of Israel*. Retrieved from http://blogs.timesofisrael.com/humor-me-heal-me/?utm_source=T...5&utm_medium=e-mail&utm_term=0_abd46cec92-42267e661e-55057237

Runde, J. (2016, September 26). Why young bankers, lawyers, and consultants need emotional intelligence. *Harvard Business Review*. Retrieved from https://hbr.org/2016/09/why-young-bankers-lawyers-and-consultants-need-emotional-intelligence

Sacks, O. (1970). *The man who mistook his wife for a hat and other clinical tales*. New York: Harper & Row.

Sacks, O. (1973). *Awakenings*. London: Duckworth & Co.

Saint Jacques, A. (2017, March 30). Survey of US physicians indicates they are overwhelmingly satisfied with their career choices. *MDLinx*. Retrieved from https://www.mdlinx.com/internal-medicine/article/781

Scott, P. J. (2016, April 16). Opioid reliance: One of the great mistakes in medical history. *Star Tribune.* Retrieved from http://www.startribune.com/reliance-on-opioids-one-of-the-greatest-mistake-in-medical-history/375906361/

Scheffler, R. M. & Glied, S. (2016, May 2). States can contain health care costs. Here's how. *The New York Times.* Retrieved from https://www.nytimes.com/2016/05/03/opinion/the-way-to-contain-health-care-costs.html

Schoenberg, E. (2016). ICD10 Consult (Version 8.0.5.) [Mobile application software].

Sergay, S. M. (2009, October 13). Doctoring 2009: Embracing the challenge. *Neurology, 73,* 1234-1239.

Serrat, O. (2009, February). The five whys technique. *Knowledge Solutions, a publication of Asian Development Bank.* Retrieved from https://www.adb.org/sites/default/files/publication/27641/five-whys-technique.pdf

Shah, A. (2015, October 28). Mediterranean diet may protect against age-related brain atrophy, dementia, new study shows. *Star Tribune.* Retrieved from http://www.startribune.com/mediterranean-diet-may-protect-against-age-related-brain-atrophy-dementia-new-study-shows/337984131/

Shah, A. (2016, February 22). 'Concussion' doctor played by Will Smith tackled CTE in football players head-on. *Star Tribune.* Retrieved from http://www.startribune.com/concussion-doctor-played-by-will-smith-tackled-cte-in-football-players-head-on/369467532/

Simmons, Z. (2015, December 8). The theory of everything: The extraordinary and the ordinary. *Neurology, 85*(23), 2079-2080.

Span, P. (2016, February 12). In palliative care, comfort is the top priority. *The New York Times.* Retrieved from https://www.nytimes.com/2016/02/16/health/in-palliative-care-comfort-is-the-top-priority.html

Stack, S. J. (2016, February 17). A call to action: Physicians must turn the tide of the opioid epidemic. *AMA Wire Alert.* Retrieved from https://wire.ama-assn.org/ama-news/call-action-physicians-must-turn-tide-opioid-epidemic

Walljasper, J. (2015, May 23). Blue Zones project helped Albert Lea, Minn., find the benefits of walking. *Star Tribune.* Retrieved from http://www.startribune.com/blue-zones-project-helped-albert-lea-minn-find-the-benefits-of-walking/304823171/

Wood, D. (2016, March). A new ecosystem for health. *Minnesota Physician, XXIX*(12), 14-15.

Wurzer, C. (Producer and Host). (December 6, 2011-2016, April 8). *Living while dying: An ALS story* [Audio podcast]. Retrieved from https://www.mprnews.org/topic/living-with-als

APPENDIX

Announcement to Neurological Associates of St. Paul (NASP) of Retirement (September 29, 2015):

It is time. As I have told our president, Nadeem, in writing, 2015 will be my last year at NASP. I love this group. It has been a wonderful run, but all good things must come to an end.

My professional career has been shared with a group of smart, hardworking, and ethical doctors, nurses, and staff who really care about our patients. I could have asked for nothing more. I leave with no doubts that our group is in good hands, and is positioned well to prosper. In addition, the future of neurology is bright. I'm confident that each of you will practice medicine as the future promises exciting and meaningful breakthroughs for our patients.

Please do not misunderstand my telling you today. I am announcing today to be able to plan a meaningful transition. I plan no tapering off. I plan no 'lame duck' behavior during my last three months at NASP. I hope to see as many patients as possible to convince them and their physicians (our referral sources) to stay with Neurological Associates. I plan to keep working at the same pace, doing the same hospital coverage, and continue to represent our group at as many hospital meetings as I can until the end of the year.

Thanks a lot and carry on.

Paul

Letter to my patients:

Dear patients of Dr. Paul Schanfield at Neurological Associates of St. Paul,

We would like to announce that after 40 years of practice with our offices, Dr. Paul Schanfield has decided to retire at the end of the calendar year 2015. He will continue to teach in the Twin Cities, as he is a Clinical Professor of Neurology at the University of Minnesota. He has also begun writing a book that will highlight what his patients have taught him about life, family, aging, and illness. The book will outline his view of the current state of medicine, his approach to the clinical practice of neurology, and his teaching philosophy.

Thank you very much for your confidence in our physicians and staff at Neurological Associates of St. Paul. We hope to smoothly transition his patients to our neurologists. If you have any questions or comments, do not hesitate to call Patty Dress, his nurse, or Stacy Fairbanks, his secretary. You may also at any time refer to our website at www.neurostpaul.com for details about our physicians.

Sincerely,

The Staff and Physicians of Neurological Associates of St. Paul

My farewell speech to the Neurology ICU staff, St Joseph's Hospital ward 5100 retirement (December 23, 2015):

We know that humor can be a defense mechanism for patients with health problems—sometimes healthy and sometimes not. We know that a positive attitude, often sprinkled with humor, can help in healing. We know, whether we admit it or not, that an amiable patient often gets better care. We know, if we stopped running around for a moment and thought about it, that humor in medicine comes from significant and intimate patient/doctor or patient/nurse interaction. We know that humor in medicine enriches the life of the doctor and the nurse, besides enhancing the chances that the patient will have a better outcome.

We know that the bedrock of good medical care is effective and humane 1:1 interaction with our patients, as individual human beings with a medical problem, not as a medical problem. The best medical care is not for "a Subarachnoid Hemorrhage in room 5144 and a Subdural Hematoma in room 5126." We know that protocols and cookbook checklists help avoid preventable mistakes, but they are not what defines truly wonderful healthcare.

Let me remind you of a few patient interactions that I recall:

- A guy told me that he now takes his pills in a shot glass, because his wife won't allow anything else in it any more.
- We had a man who had TGA, Transient Global Amnesia, here who recovered. When I saw them in the clinic, his wife agreed that his memory was fine, but he still had no common sense.
- I overheard one of our nurses chide a patient who had pulled out his Foley, "If you pull out your Foley again, you will leave here with your voice two octaves higher, I assure you."
- I walked into a room here to find an elderly, forgetful patient intently watching TV. However, it was not on.
- A 78-year-old woman was stopped by a patrol officer for eradicate driving and asked to see her license. She responded exasperatedly: "You guys should really make up your mind, officer; last week one of your partners took it away from me."
- Physician banter I overheard in the doc's lounge: "Interesting case: Don't know the diagnosis; don't know the correct treatment; fortunately, he is not my patient."
- Exceptional patient care may begin with a phone call. One of our secretaries recently answered the phone while staring at a picture of her young son, who she adores, "How may I love you today?"

I want to thank you all for doing what you do. Your jobs are challenging and the work difficult. Besides all the stresses of hospital nursing that exist today, our neuro patients may have diseases that can rob them of their intellect and/or their personality. In other words, the diseases we deal with may change the very essence of what makes a person unique. This can make our job even more emotionally draining and can lead to "burnout." Please continue to focus on those truly human moments during the day that enrich your experience.

I will miss being here with you, but I want to hear your stories. You can find me on LinkedIn. Please keep in touch. "Me . . . we . . . now."

ACKNOWLEDGMENTS

Throughout forty years of practicing medicine as clinical neurologist, I saved patient quotes and short vignettes. This store of memories became the foundation of this book, initially envisioned as a cute "coffee table book" filled with these stories. My family and my friend-turned-writing-coach, Paul Bernabei, encouraged me to weave the quotes into a full-length book, providing context for the patient experiences. This allowed me to share my philosophy of practicing and teaching clinical medicine, while critiquing today's healthcare system.

It is impossible to appropriately thank Paul Bernabei, who has spent countless hours for more than three years guiding me through this fascinating project. Thank you, Paul. I would also like to thank his wife, Paula, who allowed him to spend so much time and energy on my behalf.

The support and guidance of my family has been absolutely amazing. Their encouragement, wise counsel, and commitment to editing have been incredible. Thank you to my amazing wife, Karen, who has spent countless hours on this project. Thank you to my daughter Mara, son Adam, and my daughter-in-law Allison, who have been enthusiastic boosters and provided wise counsel.

Mara also introduced me to Brian and Scott Neville. Through an in depth email correspondence concerning the American healthcare system, Brian, a DPT* and a current PhD student, helped crystallize my critique of the system. His brother, Scott, a technical writer, provided valuable editing of the manuscript. Scott then referred me to George Stevens, of Advantage Media Group/Forbes Books, to design the cover and provide valuable publishing guidance.

It certainly took a village. This creative nonfiction project utilized the technical editing skills of Priscilla Mizell, the formatting expertise of Tim Parlin, the photography creativity of Ellie Leonardsmith Photography, and the guidance of Becky Schierman, MPH, one of the Senior Directors of the American Academy of Neurology. Three physicians, Tim Rumsey, MD (*Pictures From a Trip*), Phillip Peterson, MD (*Get Inside Your Doctor's Head*) and Scott Jensen, MD (*Relationship MATTERS: The Foundation of Medical Care Is Fracturing*) shared their book publishing experiences with me.

Long and in depth discussions with my good friend Michael Neren, MD, MBA coherently and dramatically shaped my views on today's healthcare system. Thank you, Mike. Once my ideas were written down, a close friend, Tom Kenyon, read the manuscript multiple times, suggesting a mere 600+ edits. A special thank you to David Anderson, MD and Frank Cerra, MD for reading earlier versions of the manuscript and providing me with valuable suggestions and the testimonials on the back cover.

* DPT is a Doctor of Physical Therapy